A FUTURE WITH HOPE

An Inspiring Guide to Overcoming Diabetes

BASED ON MY TRANSPARENT
LIFE AS A DIABETIC

Carl S. Armato

A Future With Hope
by Carl S. Armato

For information, contact Novant Health, 2085 Frontis Plaza Blvd., Winston-Salem, NC 27103.

FIRST EDITION

ISBN 978-0-692-15314-7

Acknowledgments

This book would not be possible without the support of my family, physicians and colleagues who have been my lifeline in my journey with diabetes.

I thank my physicians who taught me at an early age how to partner for success. This strong partnership started with my pediatrician, Carmen Posada, MD, who helped me and my family understand the disease and gave us the confidence to overcome any challenges diabetes put in our way. I'd like to thank my Novant Health physicians who have always been more than just my physicians, but who have also become my friends and colleagues: David Cook, Ophelia Garmon-Brown, Richard Kleinmann, John Pasquini, John Phipps, Ed Shoaf and Adam Spitz. I could not be the leader I am today without your support and partnership. To my colleagues and executive team members at Novant Health, thank you for everything you do to help me and all of our patients overcome challenges.

I appreciate my extended support system, which over the years has included my maternal grandparents, aunts, uncles and cousins who were there to provide help for my parents and love for me and my brothers.

I also want to thank my parents, Lucien and Leona Armato, whose unconditional love, support and encouragement made me the man I am today. They taught me that diabetes is just a part of who I am, but it in no way needs to define who I could be. They ensured that I start every day thinking of how I can help others instead of focusing on myself. That philosophy has allowed me to grow into a leader of a tremendous team of caregivers who provide remarkable care to patients every day.

My mother deserves a special thank you for learning how to care for a child with type 1 diabetes, for having the courage to ensure I had a healthy and normal childhood and for giving me the faith to believe I could thrive.

My brothers, Lenny and John, were the first people at my side if I ever needed anything but never treated me like I was fragile. We give each other a hard time, as brothers do, and I appreciate them more than they will ever understand. I'm also grateful to my father-in-law, Gus "Papa G" Guzzino, who became one of my biggest supporters after my dad passed away, and to my mother-in-law, Lula "Mama Lou" Guzzino, who continues to be a wonderful supporter.

Thanks also to my children, Carly, John and Tyler, who inspire me every day. They grew up knowing that I may need their help in a moment's notice, and that was their "normal." They have grown into amazing adults who have compassion for all people and respect those who have difficult hardships. I am incredibly proud of each one of them and the unique talents they are each offering the world. Their accomplishments make me prouder than anything I have ever done.

To the love of my life, Christi, I thank you and appreciate you every day. You have dedicated yourself to me and our family, and I am forever grateful. You have saved my life in many ways, on numerous occasions; this book is mostly dedicated to you because, let's face it, I wouldn't be the man I am today without your love, perseverance and commitment. Your loving support is the foundation for all of our success. I will love you forever.

To anyone living with diabetes or loving someone who is, I hope you enjoy reading this book. May it give you faith that you can do anything you want with your life and convince you that this disease does not need to get in your way. I hope this book also gives you some tips on managing situations for success and helps you refuse to be limited by any challenge you face in the future. I wish you a future of health, success and happiness.

Contents

Introduction

Carl Armato and I started together at Novant Health in 1998. My first job after completing my training in endocrinology was at Novant Health and Carl was one of my first patients. For seven years I was privileged to be his doctor. Over the last 20 years he has also been a colleague, a friend, a partner and now my boss. I have had a unique lens into Carl's world and a great opportunity to observe and admire his approach to living a full life with diabetes. His attitude, discipline, intellect, faith, work ethic and vision have helped him achieve amazing things personally and professionally.

I have cared for hundreds of patients who were diagnosed with diabetes as children and Carl's diagnosis at age 18 months is a common story for type 1 diabetes. It is not common for someone to live more than 50 years with diabetes and to maintain excellent health, avoid all complications and remain active. Some of that can be attributed to good fortune, or genes, or other factors for which Carl cannot take credit. However, Carl has done all of the things within his power that have enabled him to live life on his own terms.

I think Carl is as good as or better than anyone I've seen at managing diabetes. He is the gold medal winner in consistency of effort and willingness to do all the things required – count carbohydrates, check his blood sugar a lot, record it, share the data with his physician, keep his office visits and lab appointments, and more.

And he's smart. Carl's not a doctor, but I have learned so much more from him than he has learned from me. He is a very passionate person, very engaged with everything he does, but he has the ability to step outside of himself and make observations that are really helpful. He shares ideas about his experience as a diabetic that are so insightful that I say that partnering with someone as motivated as Carl is what keeps me doing this. Being a physician to Carl is like coaching a high-performing athlete; it's far more about what he does than what I do.

I have never asked him why he cares so much. It wasn't until after I'd been his doctor awhile that I came to understand how exceptional his motivation as a child was, how committed he was to a life where, through sheer force of will, diabetes was not going to get in his way. I respect Carl for a lot of things, and I am in awe of his long-term discipline and commitment. What truly mystifies me, though, is his attitude. He doesn't seem to have any "Why me?" moments. I'm actually surprised he doesn't have more of a chip on his shoulder. I'm accustomed to hearing from patients about managing their disease, "This is too hard. I'm so tired of doing it all." It's almost weird that I've never heard a word from Carl about the issue of navigating through the hard feelings associated with the disease. He's always hardworking and goal oriented, and he doesn't beat himself up when things don't go well.

Many patients' feelings about themselves can be tied to their blood sugar readings. They give themselves a grade when they take it: Their esteem goes up if it's normal, but they feel bad about themselves when it's high. That is such a difficult mindset to be in because it creates a huge disincentive to monitoring blood sugar. Carl never personalizes a high blood sugar reading as if it's something he's done wrong; rather, he sees it as an opportunity to make an adjustment.

Carl appears to manage his diabetes around the philosophy that *knowledge is power.* When some people are diagnosed with a chronic illness or serious medical condition, many of them live in denial. One way of doing that is to never embrace the need to learn about the disease. If they don't learn about it, acknowledge it or address it, maybe it will go away. Carl never did that. He has continued to learn about all aspects of diabetes and its treatment. He has been willing to embrace evolving technology and now has a Bluetooth glucose sensor that communicates with his insulin pump, allowing it to make adjustments in his insulin delivery without him having to initiate them.

Now he can have something that all of us take for granted but that he has almost never experienced: an uninterrupted night's sleep. For decades he awakened in the night to check his blood sugar. Now he can rely on the glucose sensor and the insulin pump to keep things stable overnight. Those of us who experience Carl's boundless energy have mixed feelings about him getting better sleep as we aren't sure how much more energy we can handle.

Part of Carl's story is that he has always had people around him who were willing to support him and he has been willing to allow that to happen. Like many patients with a long history of diabetes, Carl has had challenges with hypoglycemic unawareness. In these moments, he does not have the typical symptoms associated with low blood sugar and must rely on others to help him detect the problem and sometimes to help him make sure he gets his blood sugar level back up. When I first met Carl, his mom was still calling him every morning to make sure he made it through the night without any problems.

His willingness to transition to an insulin pump and to conscientiously monitor his blood sugar level afforded him some relief from the low blood sugar levels that had been occurring too frequently. When I first met Carl's mom, at a Juvenile Diabetes Research Foundation fundraiser, she hugged me and thanked me for helping Carl to get on a pump. Perhaps five years ago, Carl's wife, Christi, stopped me and tearfully thanked me for encouraging Carl to start using an insulin pump many years ago. These are only small examples of the support that Carl has had.

There are challenges for people with diabetes and for the people who want to support them. Often, people with diabetes may feel like they are constantly being monitored to make sure they are eating well and making good food choices. Imagine if you indulged in a piece of candy and you saw judgment in the eyes of people who are trying to be helpful. Carl has managed to navigate this with his family and those close to him.

Although I have heard Carl refer to himself as a diabetic, he is not defined by his disease. It is a very real and ever-present part of his life, but it isn't his life. For many years, I never spoke of Carl's diabetes to anyone because I had not heard him share this with others. His privacy meant that others would see his work and not focus on his disease. There have always been a few people close to him who were aware of his diabetes so that we could offer support when needed, including being on the lookout for symptoms of low blood sugar.

Carl's decision to share his story with 26,000 team members at Novant Health, and therefore with the world, showed incredible vulnerability and courage. Sharing his story was not about him, even though it dramatically changed how his team viewed him. He was no longer just the larger-than-life, charismatic, visionary leader. He was also someone with a significant daily challenge that he has tackled with grace for his entire life. Furthermore, it provided a lens into his heart for people, for patients, for those who meet their challenges daily.

Another aspect of his sharing was to remind people that there are important things that we all need to do to live a healthy life. Certainly there are a number of things that Carl has to do, from managing his pump, to checking his blood sugar level, to counting carbohydrates, to being always ready to address an unexpected situation. Yet his emphasis was on his more basic need to make healthy choices, to eat right, to exercise and to relieve stress. He demonstrated the need for family and friends and the importance of supporting one another. In his sharing and in his self-care, he serves as an incredible role model for our team.

Carl's life has spanned a long history in the treatment of diabetes. Although his diagnosis came at a time when a few insulins were available, glucose monitoring was not possible and there was a poor understanding of what was necessary to live well with diabetes. Carl managed his diabetes through the years of innovation and discovery with new insulins, amazing advancements in glucose monitoring and now remarkable insulin delivery systems.

In his effort to continue to live vigorously, he is attached to devices around the clock and continues to just figure it out, not accepting diabetes or its treatment as something that will stand in his way.

The privilege of being his doctor has afforded me great insights into diabetes and people who navigate it in their daily lives. Beyond that, I have worked to support Carl in his leadership of the health system. Carl has invited me and other physicians to partner with him in the strategy and operations of our health system. He understands that physicians have a unique perspective, education, training and experience that are invaluable. What we observe in Carl is something very special. He has a life experience that allows him to empathize with anyone who has had suffering or significant health challenges. He can easily say, "I know what it feels like to wake up each day and to still have diabetes, to still have to monitor blood sugar, to watch what I eat, to acknowledge fear and anxiety." To really care for people in a trusting environment, you must have vulnerability and empathy. Carl has modeled that for all of us. Because he understands what it's like to be a patient with a chronic condition, he is a compassionate leader in healthcare.

Lastly, we are setting an aspirational vision at Novant Health as it relates to caring for people with diabetes. We're not just trying to be pretty good. By the year 2020 we will be the premier health system in taking care of people with diabetes. Only knowing and working with Carl has enabled me to make such a bold statement.

– John Phipps, MD

CHAPTER ONE

DIAGNOSED: PROCESSING THE NEWS

"

"You must take
personal responsibility.
You cannot change the
circumstances, the
seasons, or the wind,
but you can
change yourself."

— *Jim Rohn,*
American entrepreneur and
motivational speaker

"OK, so I'm a diabetic." The teen was trying to sound casual, but it was evident that he was collecting his courage after walking up to me in the crowded hall. For both of us, the place seemed to fall silent. "I hear a lot of stuff at these meetings," he went on, "about how so many things can go wrong. So, what's the point?"

I had presented a talk to an audience of young people diagnosed with diabetes and their parents; my subject was, as usual, the safety precautions to be taken by diabetics and their families. Afterward, I was approached by the boy's parents, and I'd just finished talking with them when he walked up. Most of his parents' questions had been of a technical nature, but this question from him sounded almost accusatory. The boy and I looked at each other; his parents and siblings waited. I paused a moment, nodding, and repeated his last words as a statement. "What's the point."

"Right," he said. "I don't get what the big deal is about taking care of myself, if I'm gonna die soon anyway!"

The family's eyes were on me now. The faces of his mom, dad, brother and sister showed they were hoping I had the right answer. I knew my questioner was scared to death, and I knew exactly what that fear felt like.

This was a courageous kid. My heart went out to him.

"I've certainly heard your question before," I acknowledged. "Fact is, I used to ask it myself, before I was your age – and since then sometimes, too. You're wondering why you should go to all the trouble of making sure you're healthy every day, right?"

"Well . . . ," he said.

"A friend of mine recently asked me that question," I continued. "A guy about your age. He couldn't see going through all the self-care stuff, either. So I changed the subject. I asked him if he played sports. So, I'll ask you that."

"I play basketball."

"That's great. My friend told me he was a forward on his school basketball team, and they were in the playoffs. I said, 'Great. I played baseball myself, and when I had an important game coming up, like you I knew I needed to be the best I could be. That meant that in order to go all out I needed to have my blood sugar under control, make sure I hadn't eaten too much, and things like that.' So I guess that's my answer to you. If you're serious about playing basketball – or anything else you want to do or be a part of – I'm sure you want to beat the odds against diabetes, like I did."

The youngster's tone was different when he asked, "So, when did you find out you were a diabetic?"

I smiled. "I might be kind of a poster boy for that. I was 18 months old." I let that sink in, then added, "I'm 52 now." I could feel his parents' and siblings' relief beginning to set in. "My mom was worried; she told my pediatrician how I was drinking a lot of water and crying all night. But he always told her she worried too much. Lucky for me, that pediatrician was out of town when Mom saw some blood and took me to our family doctor. When he ran a blood test, the doc said I probably would have died the next day, just dropping into a coma without anyone ever realizing what was happening."

I shot a look at my questioner. "That's pretty much the way you'll go out, too, if you don't take care of yourself."

"Anyway," I went on, "I got my first insulin shot that night, as a toddler. Since then, for more than five decades, I've been learning how to live my life as a diabetic – refusing to believe I was going to die before I was a teenager or go blind in my 20s; refusing to buy into the notion that I couldn't be a champion tennis player or an all-star shortstop; refusing to believe I couldn't fall in love, marry and have a wonderful family; and refusing to think I could never be a successful professional, just because of diabetes."

The kid had moved closer to me; I noticed the change in his eyes.

"So that's my one-word answer to your question," I told him.

"What?" he said.

"Refuse, refuse, refuse. Can you do that?"

"Yes, sir," he replied, smiling suddenly.

After the hope settled in, I said, "But I want to make one point really clear, my friend, to you and your family. So, are you listening? You've got to support your supporters. I'm no hero. The heroes in my life are my parents and the people who supported me. Those are your heroes, too. They're the ones who watch and make sure you're OK, so they're the ones to listen to. You need to support your supporters: love them, appreciate them and, above all, listen to them. And do it like your life depends on it."

I participate in a few of these meetings a year, most of which are sponsored by the American Diabetes Association. I also invite teens and their families into my home, not to preach to them but to listen as they voice their fears or concerns, and to try to be of help. I want to make them the stars of the get-together. I know I have to earn my response to each question they ask, comment they make or story they tell.

Listening is the key. Underneath every question or story I hear from young diabetics or their parents, fear is lurking. For people with diabetes, the often-heard comment "It's not a matter of life or death" has no place. Somehow, through the way they've taught me to listen to them, I've learned to frame my message of due diligence in a way that gets through to them. It's more than a warning; it's a campaign. It's war, and you fight if you want to survive.

As I told the audience that night, it started very early for me. In the mid 1960s, life as a toddler with diabetes in my hometown of Patterson, on the Gulf Coast in rural Louisiana, was not easy. My parents, Lucien and Leona Armato, were told that I was the youngest child ever to be diagnosed with diabetes in St. Mary Parish. As a 24-year-old mother of two boys, my mom was scared. My brother, Lenny, was not even 3 years old yet, and now my mom had an 18-month-old with diabetes. She had no idea how to take care of me.

The day after my diagnosis, my parents took me to Ochsner Hospital in New Orleans, where – fortunately for my parents and for me – I became the young patient of Carmen Posada, MD. She was not a pediatric endocrinologist. I don't even know if such a specialty existed in 1966. But Dr. Posada was a pediatrician with a real understanding of and interest in endocrinology for type 1 diabetes.

The doctor was very aggressive with the insulin and worked hard to get my blood sugar level down. My parents finally were able to take me back to Patterson, but Dr. Posada wanted to see me often. So every month Mom and I made the 90-minute drive to New Orleans until my blood sugar levels were consistently under control. I continued to see Dr. Posada once a year until I was a teenager.

Parents as Partners

Diabetes affects everyone around you. Whether you're dealing with a baby who has no understanding of what is happening or with an older child, it's a 24-hours-a-day, seven-days-a-week disease.

Mom and Dad had a long talk after they brought me home from New Orleans. It was the kind of talk all parents of children with diabetes need to have, earlier rather than later.

"We didn't see this coming, Leona," my dad said, "but it's our job. We are the ones with the responsibility to take care of Carl until he's able to do it himself."

"I agree, of course," my mother said, tearfully. "I'm with you in it, honey, all the way."

"So, it's a pact. We're partners in this."

I can imagine their eyes shining as they made that agreement. It was a turning point. From then on, Mom told me, it was a partnership, and no one was left out. Dad, Mom, Lenny and my younger brother, John, who arrived five years later – the whole family adopted the new diet and lifestyle that was necessary for me, their diabetic family member, to survive and thrive. And they stuck to it. I am so proud of them. They are truly my heroes.

Mom especially did not have it easy partnering with me to keep the disease in check while I was a child. Thankfully, home treatment technology has advanced a good deal since the 1960s. Whereas today we have glucometers to measure blood sugar and pumps to automatically inject insulin, back then you couldn't check your blood sugar at home. The best you could do was test your urine to see how much sugar had spilled out of your blood system and into your waste water. This was a very primitive way of measuring your success. Visiting the doctor every month for a single blood test wasn't much better because it provided only a snapshot, not an overview.

Even so, these were the tools and methods my mom had at her disposal 50 years ago. Following my diagnosis, she and Dad had vowed to care for me and monitor my diabetes until I could do it myself, and her part in the campaign meant she'd need to make changes to our daily life – changes that unnerved her at first but that soon helped her understand and manage the disease for me.

'Unless You Know the Disease'

While the parents of most kids Carl's age were just trying to potty train their young ones, my young son and I had a different routine.

First thing every morning I would wake Carl up, get him to the bathroom and have him empty his bladder. Then I'd make breakfast or do other things, waiting a suitable time for fresh urine to build up so he could urinate again. I'd get him to urinate into a small orange plastic cup; and going to my little chemistry set, I'd take out a small test tube and pour the urine into it. I would add a tablet and, just like a chemist, examine the color to decide whether the mixture showed he had sugar in his blood.

Next came the part I dreaded. I was always scared of needles. But Dr. Posada had me give myself a shot in my leg, with water, to show me that it didn't hurt. Then she had me practice with an orange. Had it not been for her, we would have had a rough time. You've got to know the disease. If you don't know what's happening, you can't help a child that young.

Each morning after testing the sugar in Carl's urine I would give him a fixed dosage of insulin prescribed by the physician. Finally I would record the amount of sugar in a journal, which I would show to the doctor at our next visit. She would read my notes and adjust the insulin intake as she thought necessary. Dr. Posada told me, "You can't treat him or take care of him unless you know the disease." The doctor met with me for three weeks, twice a day – morning and afternoon – and taught me what I needed to do, and what I needed to know.

– *Leona Armato*

—— *Consider this* ——

REFUSE
to let
DIABETES
DEPRIVE YOU OF
hope or success.

THE MORE YOU
exercise control
OVER DIABETES,
the less it has control
OVER YOU.

'Help Us to Help Them All We Can'

Every morning when my dad woke up, as his feet hit the floor at his bedside, he would ask God for someone he could help. And God sent a lot of people to him.

"My name is Phil Blaney, and I'm an exterminator. I got to know Lucien Armato when I was hired to spray for bugs at the bank where he worked. I was having my lunch outside and Lucien came and sat down and talked with me. In my business, people don't tend to do that, but Lucien was as friendly as he could be. He kept coming back, or greeting me when he would see me. He never forgot my name. Lucien was one of those people who take a genuine interest in you. And they're rare."

As the man sat down, I looked at my mother sitting next to me in the church pew. She was shaking her head in wonder. I think she was as amazed as I was that so many people had shown up for my dad's wake and funeral.

Next up was a couple. The wife spoke. "We've had so many good times as a family in our trailer," she began. "We didn't know how we would be able to finance it, but –" She stopped and broke down; her husband put his arm around her and waited. "But Lucien Armato made it possible. He went out of his way to arrange our loan. So many times," again she paused and dabbed at her nose, "when we were on the road on one of our trips, we thought of him."

"We often said we should have had a picture of Lucien up in the trailer," her husband added. "Such a kind man. Such a kind man."

I recognized the next individual who stood up.

He was our handyman, Andrew. "I can't add too much. You all know what a special person Mr. Armato was. I just wanted to honor him. I got to know him pretty well, working around you-all's place. He always treated me as a real friend," he remarked.

Another individual spoke up. "Mr. Armato was a help to us in getting some of the medications we needed for our father. Your father was a remarkable man; he was always trying to help us. We will miss him."

I looked around the funeral home and church. It was fuller than it was some Sundays for Mass. All these people, many of whom I didn't know, had shown up at my dad's funeral. It made me so proud of my father.

Another man noted, "I've been listening to how many of you Lucien Armato helped to buy your homes. I was one of those. I know you know this, but in a way any bank's loan officer could help you get a house. It was the way Lucien Armato did it, the care he took to get you the best rate, and just the careful way he went about it. I felt he was as happy to see me get my new home as I was."

There were many people who wanted to add a word about my father. With each one I felt more and more honored to be his son. After the service, so many people lined up to shake Mom's hand or give her a hug that it was quite a long time before we could leave the funeral home and church. Many people greeted my brothers and me, too. Everyone was so kind.

Driving home, as Mom kept talking to Lenny, John and me about the service, I chimed in, "Do you remember the lady who said that God sent an angel to help her, and it was Dad?" Everyone exclaimed at that;

we had all been moved by it. "Well," I continued, "I feel like God sent Dad to help me."

My dad had a tough life. He lost his father when he was 10, and his mother died when he was 12. With no father or mother, he went from relative to relative, eventually living with his older sister. I often wondered how somebody who grew up without a dime and without parents, who moved from family to family, eventually went to college and built a family like ours.

And yet I know the answer. It was his deep faith in God. Through his belief in Christ and in prayer, he found the hope to completely change the unfortunate life he had as a child into what he wanted it to be for himself and his family. By the time I came along, the second of his three sons, and was diagnosed at 18 months with a disease many people at the time considered to be a killer, Dad had already made himself into an overcomer, a conqueror of difficulties. He demonstrated that same hope for me and our family that had brought him through life.

I can hear him today, his rich baritone voice ringing as he was giving encouragement to someone. "No matter what problems you have," he would say, "or what cards you've been dealt, just apply yourself as best you can and then do the best with what you have."

With that optimistic outlook and strong faith in God, my father and mother and my two brothers together became my primary support system as I grew up and learned how to become a diabetes survivor. As the spiritual backbone of our family, Dad's faith and optimism were on hand countless times to ease our fears and troubles. Besides being the primary provider, one of his key roles was to guide us spiritually.

"You guys all brushed your teeth?" he'd ask.

"Yeah, Dad." "Yeah." "Yes, sir," we'd reply.

"OK, let's get down and do it."

As I closed my eyes, my father's warm presence covered me like a cozy blanket. My brothers and I loved this time each night, with Dad watching over us as we said our prayers at bedtime. It was his quiet way of spreading his spiritual faith and hope to us. After a silence during which we were supposed to pray silently, his quiet voice would fill the room with its humble entreaties. "Lord, help Lenny, Carl and John with their studies. Please allow the talents you have given them to come to life. And thank you so much for how well Carl is doing with his diabetes. Lord, please continue to bless our family. And don't forget how grateful Leona and I are for giving us such great boys. Help us to help them all we can."

When a pause came, we boys would be ready to get up off of our knees and into bed, but we'd learned to wait. Sure enough, there was more. "God, you know that Tommy Lindstrom down the street needs your help, and we pray for him. And Uncle Vincent is sick and needs your help, too, Lord."

Another pause. Then: "Amen."

Indeed, God sent a lot of people to Dad. But the distinct feeling I get, having grown from childhood to young adulthood under Dad's guidance, is that the Lord sent Dad to me.

As much as Mom was a pivotal partner in managing

the day-to-day health of her diabetic child, Dad's steady faith and encouragement set the tone for accepting the disease in stride. Following his lead, I learned to view the diagnosis as an opportunity to exercise control over the diabetes rather than allowing diabetes to exercise control over me.

Of course, at the time, I was much too young to understand the implications of this diagnosis to my long-term health, if the disease went unmanaged. My parents understood, though. Even so, they refused to accept the negatives as certainties. Instead, the diagnosis served as a launching point for a positive campaign my whole family has joined – to create a full and active lifestyle that refuses to let diabetes deprive us of success or happiness.

So really, when I speak to people – especially young people – grappling with their diagnosis, it's not my advice I offer. It's the advice of family members who've shaped me, supported me and never allowed diabetes to place limits on me. But it's good advice, all the same.

Refuse.

CHAPTER TWO

SUPPORT: A CRUCIAL FOUNDATION

"

"Choose to *focus* your time, energy and conversation around people who *inspire* you, support you and help you to *grow* you into your happiest, strongest, wisest self."

———————

– Karen Salmansohn,
Author and relationship expert

What anyone with diabetes soon learns is that you can't do this alone; a good, steady support system, even if it's one or two people, is like the breath of life. If you're lucky, you find this out before you have a series of crises. If your low blood sugar level is causing you to lose the ability to think clearly, and a member of your regular support cadre isn't around, then you need another skill. It's the skill of overcoming your ego – the part of you that doesn't want to acknowledge you're in trouble, that tries to somehow solve the issue without anyone knowing.

I am calling that ability to overcome your pride or embarrassment or fierce self-sufficiency a skill because it means you've learned to handle your vulnerability as part of your set of self-care abilities. Having the presence of mind to tell yourself when the chips are down (by which I mean *before* the chips are down, of course) can be a lifesaving strategy. There is no shame – in fact, there is *wisdom* – in telling yourself, "I have to let these people help me." It's not easy to do, especially if you're among strangers and only half-conscious that you're doing it.

Once, on a break during a conference, I went into the hotel lobby. There I saw a middle-aged guy who wasn't saying much but was obviously in some confusion. The front desk clerk was trying to get him to express what he needed. It was winter outside, but I noticed a cold sweat running down the man's face. As I watched him, I noticed that although he had lost the ability to communicate clearly, he was rejecting the help being offered.

Realizing he was in a stupor, I ran to the break area, got an orange juice and a sweet croissant and brought them to the man. For some reason he trusted me. He sat down, ate the food, drank the juice and recovered completely in 15 minutes. He told me he was an attorney and admitted he was having an insulin reaction. I told him I had type 1 diabetes, which was how I knew he'd been in trouble. The point here is twofold: First, people with diabetes can be their own best or worst supporter, depending on how willing they are to ask for or accept help. Second, if you're a support person, sometimes your job is to figure out how to give help to a person who is refusing it.

Another story involves a person I knew with type 2 diabetes who recently passed away. Years ago he'd started taking insulin, but he wasn't taking care of himself where his diet was concerned. I bought a glucometer (a blood glucose-measuring device that can be purchased at a drugstore) and gave it to him one day when I saw him in a parking lot. While he was thanking me for it, he told me that the previous day he'd been driving along a road when he'd had an insulin reaction. "I pulled over and sat there," he recounted, "not knowing what to do."

"Congratulations, Jack," I said, "for making it here to tell me about it."

He smiled. "Yeah, that was scary."

"So the point is," I said, "to test your blood sugar *before* getting in your car to drive any distance." I went over to my car, took out a can of Sprite and some glucose tablets and gave them to him. "Keep these in your car," I advised.

A few weeks later I saw him again, and he commented, "Carl, you saved my life. I was on the road and I got delirious again. I didn't realize where I was. But I drank the Sprite and took the pills and was able to continue."

Helping people during times like that comes naturally to me because I grew up with such a great support system of my own. Even now I often recall going into my parents' bedroom in the middle of the night with hypoglycemia, or low blood sugar. I was having an insulin reaction; when I was young, we called it "getting weak." So when I entered their bedroom and said, "I'm weak," Mom would be instantly awake; she'd get up, give me some orange juice and stay with me until I felt better. Often she would stay up with me for a couple of hours to be sure the reaction had passed.

Support Starts at Home

Mom worked at a bank during my childhood, but she was always at school activities and ballgames. She took care of us at home and made sure we – especially I – had the right food. She helped me understand the right foods to eat and the appropriate portions of food to take in. With her care in cooking, she always focused on providing an appropriate diet to keep me healthy.

The beauty of how my parents reacted to my disease is that they adjusted our whole family's lifestyle. It wasn't just an adjustment made to *my* diet. Mom cooked the same meals for the whole family. I didn't have a different plate than everyone else; we all ate the same food.

—————— *Consider this* ——————

YOU CAN'T
do this
ALONE.

The diabetic diet and approach to life became normal for all of us, not just for me. I didn't feel that I was so different. Of course, my parents made occasional exceptions for my siblings, like making cakes at birthdays, but I was always included, just with different adjustments and tweaks.

"Here's your cake, Carl," Mom would say, handing me a small slice of pound cake without icing. It was John's birthday, and even though I couldn't have a regular slice, she made sure I was included. I was never treated as an outlier. I didn't know I was so different. Even on my own birthdays, Mom had a small piece of cake without icing for me so my birthday was special.

Mom and Dad were so smart in the way they worked with me. To help with my diabetes, they had me focus on just a few concepts that I could understand at an early age. One was the importance of testing my urine for sugar content. Another was getting lots of exercise. They thought exercise would help counter anything that the disease could do because not only did it help keep my blood sugar down, but it also had a positive impact on me psychologically. "The more exercise you have," they would say, "and the more fun you have doing it, the better."

Crisis Avoidance Through Exercise

My parents had very good reasons for encouraging me to exercise. They reminded me that food, stress and hormones can raise blood sugar from the normal range (72–99 mg/dl before eating and up to 140 mg/dl after eating) and that my insulin and exercise will lower high blood sugar levels. While a person without diabetes will very seldom have a blood sugar level outside this normal range, people with diabetes can see blood sugar levels range from 40 to 300 in a typical day and will struggle each day to strike a balance that maintains this normal range.

When my blood sugar is high or begins to move above 180, I generally begin to feel sluggish, tired and hungry. As my blood sugar level rises, I also feel nauseous. High blood sugar over a longer period of time can cause organ damage. Blood sugar that remains out of control for an extended period of time can bring on diabetic ketoacidosis (DKA), coma and, rarely, death.

My parents taught me how effective insulin and exercise could be in combating the dangers of high blood sugar, but I also had to watch how much exercise I did each day. Too much exercise made my blood sugar fall to very low levels, such as 60 mg/dl and lower. This hypoglycemia is an insulin reaction that can range from mild to severe, much like its consequences, if unaddressed.

During an insulin reaction, a person with diabetes may feel very weak, begin to shake, break out in a cold sweat and even have blurred or double vision. Eventually, if low blood sugar is not treated, the person can lose consciousness and won't wake up without medical assistance. If no such assistance is provided, a diabetic could die. Fortunately, I did not have a severe insulin reaction until I was older.

The Support Cadre

As my parents learned the positive effects that exercise has on diabetes, athletics became a big part of our family life. We took walks, and when my brothers and I were older, we learned to play sports like tennis, baseball and basketball. Lenny and John learned to watch out for me and recognize signs that I needed help.

As we were all learning to deal with episodes of low blood sugar during my sporting activities, a typical scenario and a supportive exchange went something like this: Lenny walks into the baseball dugout when it's our turn to bat and asks, "Carl, are you all right? You look like you're out of it. You're not playing at the level you're capable of!"

I reply, "I'm fine, I'm fine. I'm just not on right now." Lenny looks at my glassy eyes; he knows I'm experiencing low blood sugar. He also knows I'll never admit to having an off day unless I'm having low blood sugar. He hands me a Coke and tells me, "Sit down and drink this."

I still insist I'm fine. "Just leave me alone," I tell him. Lenny gets louder. "You're not paying attention!"

"I am so!" I shout.

"Come on," Lenny urges, "we're just going to sit for a few minutes and drink this Coke so your sugar will go up."

I shake my head, but then John walks up and asks, "Hey, Carl, what's going on? What are you feeling? Do you need me to get you something to eat or another Coke?"

I think, *What's the use?* I cave.

My family often worked as a team to deliver rock-solid support in the way I needed. Later, both my brothers extended their support into our days together at college. Lenny had a dream of attending Louisiana State University in Baton Rouge, but he sacrificed it to be with me as I pursued an accounting degree at University of Southwestern Louisiana (USL), now University of Louisiana at Lafayette.

My extended support system included my maternal

grandparents, aunts, uncles and cousins who were there to provide help for my parents and love for me and my brothers. Once I was school age, my extended system of supporters grew to include teachers and counselors.

Mom has never forgotten how much Dr. Posada helped her prepare to be my caregiver. The training she received while I was hospitalized provided the foundation she needed; and if she ever had questions, the doctor was a phone call away. In fact, to this day, decades later, she and Dr. Posada are still friends and talk by phone, even though the doctor has retired.

I found out years later just how taxing it was for Mom. At one point when I was a child, my diabetes and my constant need for her care made her so nervous and anxious she told our family doctor she needed some medicine to calm her nerves. But the doctor refused to prescribe Valium for her. Instead, he told Mom she would just have to learn to live with her role in my support system. And she did, without ever relying on prescriptions.

Mom provided me with the kind of love and emotional support only a mother can give. In addition to making sure our whole family ate appropriately, she also monitored my daily insulin dosage and gave me insulin shots until I was 8 years old and could administer them myself. Mom was a remarkable caregiver for me in my early years.

Supporting Role: To Protect and Empower

Mom's support has never waned; but as I grow older I notice that it also has never lost that tinge of tentativeness about how events will affect my health. When I was offered the job as president of the Charlotte market of

Novant Health, I went home and talked to my mom and my wife, Christi, about it. Dad had passed away by then, and Mom was being her cautionary self: "Oh, honey, why would you want all that stress?"

A different reaction came from Leonard "Gus" Guzzino, Christi's dad, who had watched me grow up and deal with the disease over the years. He said, "Take the opportunity. Try it and see how it goes. I'm confident you'll deal with the stress."

I was thankful to Mr. Guzzino, but I had others around me who communicated sentiments along the lines of "Poor Carl, he has so much he has to deal with in life." This attitude can be reinforced by people who think they're looking out for you. Having people like this in your support system can pull you down into victim mode. The last thing I wanted to hear was "Poor Carl." Of course it's coming from love, but there's pity in it, too, which can drag you down.

Care providers have to ask themselves, "What kind of message am I providing?" If it's pity, it can actually make people with diabetes hide out more or accept less in life than they are capable of. But care providers who guard their words and behavior from the suggestion of pity can become an asset to a support system – a strong asset, even, if the messages carry encouragement or prompt people with diabetes to think their choices through.

My dad (for one) was this kind of care provider for me. When I was a kid, he always lifted me up to where the opportunity was and prompted me to think about how I could make myself better.

Dad had the wisdom to always point out why I was special – why the disease made me special and what it was going to help me do in life. He reminded me that having diabetes helped me understand how others with illnesses really felt and that I could use this to help others. He turned diabetes into a real positive for me. He laid the groundwork by letting me know he would be with me and together we would not let diabetes get in my way.

I remember how Mom and Dad would take me for checkups as a child – checkups that always required someone to draw blood. The nurse would come out to where my dad was waiting and say, "Well, Mr. Armato, we're going to have to call in a few people to hold him down." And Dad would say, "That will not be necessary. Carl, show them." And I would plop my arm down, big and strong.

Dad made me believe there was nothing that I could not do. I am sure that is the reason I am here today, doing what I do. I try to bring that same attitude, to help others see it in themselves. I try to get people to do things they never thought were possible because that's what I was taught.

Not an Easy Job

Dealing with my disease certainly was never easy for my family. Fortunately for me, just as Dad always found ways to help others outside our home, he decided to help me beat diabetes. He and Mom, by developing the support group that I needed, helped me learn to manage the disease and not let it always be in control of my life.

CHAPTER THREE

OWN THE DISEASE

"There is a *giant* asleep in every man. When that giant wakes, *miracles* can happen."

———————

– Frederick Faust,
American novelist

It's very natural, when you find out you have a lifelong disease, to ask *Why me?* or at least to feel somehow unfaired-against. All the victim thinking kicks in. Particularly when I was young, that inner battle went on. I tried not to show it; but in school and other places, it was difficult to see my friends not have the limits or restrictions I had.

I felt jealous of them; they didn't have to do what I had to do. They could just get up in the morning and eat what they wanted. At school lunch I would sit there eating the additional vegetables or special diabetic diet, watching the other kids eat desserts and imagining what it would be like if I could eat normally. But I had a job to do that they didn't have: taking care of myself.

"Carl, you are exasperating!" my second-grade teacher told me one day. "Here I've gone to all the trouble to give the class a treat of ice cream sandwiches, and you're holding out. You are just being stubborn!"

"But Mrs. Como, I tell you I can't eat it. It's not good for me. You can check with my mom."

Later that day the teacher called my mother, and Mom told her about my diabetes. When I got home, Mom rewarded me for taking a stand. She said I could have had a little taste of ice cream, but I still refused because I knew it was something that a person with diabetes shouldn't eat.

Mrs. Como became my friend for life. Whenever I came home from college, and even after I started my career, I would see Mrs. Como at church and get the biggest hug from her. Until she died in her 80s, she would always remind me of the determined little second-grader who refused to eat his ice cream sandwich.

For me, that day in second grade was a significant event in my life as well. From that point on, I owned my disease and took responsibility to manage my life as a diabetic. It's something all diabetics have to do.

A Serious Matter

Growing up, I had some friends who were examples of what I didn't want to do or be; some of those people are not with us today. I knew other young people with diabetes who didn't have the supportive environment I had. Consequently, they didn't develop a commitment to follow the rules, and their lives were cut short.

Given the seriousness with which my family took the disease, I was shocked at the absence of such an attitude in some of my friends with diabetes. One student in my elementary school class, Roy Ascher, was a mischievous guy who sat next to me and once put a tack on my chair. Roy really had no support system; he was virtually on his own. Though it was sad, you could see from the beginning how it wasn't going to work out for him. He was taking insulin on his own, but the important matters of seeing a doctor and following a diet just were not in place. He got into smoking and lots of things that were not good for people with diabetes.

Without a proper support system, it's even more crucial to take ownership of managing this disease. My family's support when I was young grew me into a somewhat proficient manager. Lacking that kind of support, Roy, who was left to self-manage from a young age, sometimes came up short in the area of diligence. I remember one Halloween where this looked a bit like freedom to me – freedom that stepped on my diligent, rule-following toes.

As a kid, I was never happy to see Halloween roll around. While other children would proudly collect huge bags of candy and goodies, my family would give me bananas and apples and unsalted popcorn. My brothers used to tease me when I dumped out my bag. "Hey look, Carl," they'd say. "You've got a fruit salad!"

But then when I was about 10 years old, diabetic chocolate candy bars were introduced. That year I got two whole bars from my folks! I was so excited. Then Roy Ascher showed up at our door, munching on real chocolate bars like all the other kids. So what did my dad say to me? You guessed it.

"Carl, why don't you give Roy one of your diabetic bars?"

I objected. "But Dad, he's eating regular candy!"

"Exactly. That's why he needs one of yours!"

So I gave up one of my bars. Sad to say, years later Roy died at the wheel. The disease is such a silent killer.

Another boy, younger than me, was diagnosed at 14 with type 1 diabetes. He came to me and I spent time talking to him, trying to influence him about the guiding principles. But he was very relaxed about it all. His parents told my mom that he never followed the rules like I did. He never committed to it but just went through the motions and didn't stay focused. Unfortunately, he died of kidney failure.

Mom and Dad had set such a strong foundation of support so I could thrive; over the years, I often noticed that other young people with diabetes either lacked that supportive foundation or chose not to comply and thrive in it. The observation helped me understand this about diabetes: The disease is the disease, but it's how people deal with diabetes and adapt to it that is critical to the quality of life they have – more importantly, to whether they even have a life to live.

Overcoming Self-Pity and Other Inner Battles

I remember a day when a bunch of us boys were playing ball in the backyard, taking turns trying to hit the ball over the fence. It turned out I was the only one who couldn't make it that day. I was experiencing a low blood sugar level; so, feeling weak, I went into the house. My mind was mucking around in self-pity: *Look at that. I'm the only kid who can't get the ball over the fence. Why can't I just be normal?*

Dad saw my face and knew right away what was going on. He picked me up and had me look out the window at a boy who was sitting over to the side – a friend who was disabled and had to get around on crutches. Dad said, "Look over there at Danny. Every time you feel sorry for what you've been dealt, think about how there are folks who face greater challenges than you do. Now, get your blood sugar right, and go out there and hit the ball."

I did, and I hit one over the fence.

I don't mean to imply that growing up I did not subject myself to self-pity. As a person with diabetes, you are likely to fight that self-pity all the time. When you're young, you're jealous of so-called normal kids. (It took me a number of years to understand that there's really no "normal.") Later, when you're in the work world, you're wondering if the disease will hold you back in your career. *Will others see me and think my diabetes won't allow me to handle the next promotion?* The truth is, diabetes isn't the only card in the hand you've been dealt; there's also the mentality, the inner battles that go along with it.

Dilemma: Reveal or Conceal?

As you may have guessed, people with diabetes constantly deal with the issue of who knows and who doesn't. The temptation is always there to keep it hidden, to tell no one except your inner circle. Such a decision has both good and bad points. The last thing I wanted was to have people thinking, *Poor Carl.* On the other hand, I had to be extra diligent in my self-care; if I were in an environment where no one knew I had diabetes and my blood sugar wasn't controlled, there could be consequences.

My whole life I've struggled with whether or not to tell people I have diabetes. I was afraid they would see my disease as a negative or view me as fragile. I just wanted to be treated like a regular person. Mom used to argue with me on this point often. She always wanted to tell people up front, especially at school, so she could be sure I was supported when I was away from her.

When we were proactive about acknowledging my

disease, people dealt with it in different ways. For example, when we told the cafeteria workers at school, they helped me. If I said I wanted more vegetables and fewer carbohydrates when I went through the line, right on the spot they would make those adjustments. They always kept up a relationship with me: "Here comes Carl. He's going to eat the turnip greens."

—— *Consider this* ——

It's the hand

YOU'VE BEEN DEALT–

SO PLAY IT

to win!

Of course, my teachers, like Mrs. Como, were always helpful. The guidance counselors at the schools I attended in Patterson helped me manage my disease by providing space in their file cabinets for my snacks. Whenever I felt weak and needed something sugary to manage my disease, I went to a closet in the guidance counselor's office and chose something from the file cabinet inside. The counselor had placed my Cokes and cookies there so I could access them even if he or she were absent.

Having that special arrangement was part of owning the disease and enlisting key people to help my family manage it. But I also knew not to abuse the arrangement, partly because it would violate the trust between me and my teachers or counselors, but mostly because I took managing my health seriously. I never violated a rule when it came to snacking. I didn't try to sneak food or drinks, at school or at home. Mom and Dad told me that if I wanted something, I should come to them. They knew I could have a snack, and we could exercise to deal with the food's effect on me. So there was never a need for me to hide what I was eating. Maybe that's why it struck me as a little intrusive or even irritating when well-meaning people quizzed me on my health and habits.

As I was growing up, whenever people – especially adults – learned that I had diabetes, they almost always treated me differently. Either they asked me about it ("Are you OK?"), or they constantly reminded me that I have diabetes. For example, at meals they would ask, "Are you supposed to be eating that?" That was aggravating because even when I needed sugar, people were asking me why I was eating it.

Friends my age were the exceptions. We were schoolmates in the classroom, and we played together as little kids and on teams as we grew older. To most of them, I was not Carl, the diabetic. I was just Carl. But other people's lack of knowledge about the disease was almost as burdensome as personally dealing with it; I found myself constantly having to explain why I was doing what I did. I can easily understand why some people get frustrated, give up and stop trying to manage their diabetes.

In my middle school years, one instance proved to be a turning point for me. I was the starting point guard on the middle school team. Mom worried I might have a reaction on the court, in a game or at practice, so I told the coach about my diabetes. Then I informed Mom, "You don't have to worry about anything. I have everything under control. I took care of it myself." But it didn't work out that way. As soon as I told the coach about my disease, I found I was no longer a starter. In fact, I didn't play much at all after that.

Now, I can't be too critical of that coach. He really was just trying to look out for me, but he did not understand how well I was managing my diabetes.

I went home and told Mom, "Look, I told him and now I don't play. I think he's afraid." And he was afraid. He would send me into a game for a little while, and then he'd pull me out and ask, "Are you OK? Do you need anything?"

Needless to say, when that coach left our school, I didn't tell the next coach. When he asked me why I hadn't been starting, I shrugged. We didn't have glucometers on the bench in those days, so I learned at that age to hide my disease and to manage it under the radar. Before long, I was back in the starting five. At that point in my life, in middle school, I swore that I would never again tell anybody I had diabetes.

When I told my parents I would never tell another person, they were upset that I'd made the decision because someone had responded in this way to my diabetes. They tried to figure out how to get me to understand that we still had to tell people. Until that point, Mom had always gone to talk to my teachers. She wanted to make sure that both of us had the conversation so they knew I was a diabetic, in case I needed to get up and go to my file cabinet drawer. After my experience with the coach, we stopped doing that.

"You know," I reasoned with my folks, "I'm the only one who can deal with this anyway. These people don't understand it, and they're not going to help me. So why don't you just let me have my own file cabinet of stuff? People need to know that when I have to get up and go somewhere, they just need to let me go." I was a stubborn teenager, and insistent. After I'd explained myself in this way, Mom never went against my wishes by telling people about my diabetes.

Shine Despite the Diabetes

After that turning point, the news of my diabetes was mine to reveal or conceal. Stubbornly, I didn't reveal it much. I was actually so stubborn that I committed to outperforming everybody to compensate for the disease. Under my own pressure to outdo people so that no one would recognize I had diabetes, I was the star of every team I played on. I always felt I had something to prove: being a top athlete, earning a 4.0 GPA while in graduate school. I constantly tried to prove to myself that the disease wasn't holding me back.

In fact, I kept my disease to myself almost exclusively, even after I finished college and started my career. I was concerned about whether people would hold it against me. When I interviewed for jobs, I worried about whether or not to be up front about my diabetes. Not until years later, when I was a successful professional with a wife and three children, did I change my mind and start to tell my story.

Confidence is always being tested in the lives of those with diabetes, not the least in the matter of career. If you're disease free, all things being equal you have a good shot at a challenge. But the person with diabetes thinks, *Will the disease hold me back?*

Not many people know this, but early in my career I often struggled with those victim thoughts and I didn't want others to know it. I might have talked to a few people with diabetes but I hid out from the rest, so they saw the success but not the struggle. For a long time, I didn't tell people about my diabetes except those in my inner circle. I looked the healthiest. I was the athlete. I was the heartiest in the workplace. From all outward appearances, others would never know of my diabetes, so the temptation was to hide it. My mind would run through questions that I imagine many people with this condition ask. *Are they going to pity me? Will I get weird questions about what I eat?* I constantly evaluated whether or not to tell.

Managing Self Can Motivate Others

Diabetes is a never-ending disease, every hour of every day. You can't decide to manage it one day and not the next. I began learning how to live with the disease as a child when my mother helped me pay such close attention to my diet and my father emphasized the importance of exercise. I was blessed because my parents were such good caretakers. But at some point, I instinctively knew I needed to step into that main caretaker role for myself; after all, it was *my* future, my plan for a career and family, that I was investing in.

Stepping Up To Self-Manage

My son, Carl, began to take on more responsibility for managing his diabetes as a teenager. Even in the second grade, he knew right from wrong. But after he went to a camp for children with diabetes, he learned how to take the shots. When he went on to college, he knew what he could do and what he couldn't.

Even from childhood, he was disciplined to monitor his habits to feel his best. I've often said there's no way you can tempt Carl. He tells me he wanted things for his future; he wanted to get married and have a family. Carl wanted the opportunities that others without diabetes had. So he knew he had to take care of himself.

– Leona Armato

I often tell people, "Listen to your own voice. Believe in your own know-how as manager of your diabetes. Pay no attention to what others think of you." I know that courage is nurtured and flourishes under adversity. Since that's so, I figure the disease almost gives me an "in" with those who have it. I was once with a patient with whom I felt I could say these things, and I told him, "Diabetes is a great gift, don't you think? Look how lucky we are! We have it over other people, because we're conquerors inside. Our spirit as overcomers can contribute to the world."

Of course, it isn't just people with diabetes who need uplifting. Isn't adversity what life offers? I heard a story about someone praying, "Lord, I'm having a pretty good day so far. I haven't been grumpy or snapped at anyone. And I've made no errors at work. But in a few minutes I'm going to get out of bed, and that's when I'll really need Your help." Unless they stay in bed in the morning, people typically have to overcome challenges – if not illness, then losses (pets, jobs, marriages, loved ones), habits, addictions, disappointments and a host of other things they just don't tell others about.

I've heard the advice, "Be kinder than necessary, for everyone you meet is fighting some sort of battle." The more we understand, and the more we overcome in our own lives, the more we awaken that spirit in others. Imagine how we could encourage or even inspire others who know our condition and see us thrive.

When I was younger and chose to keep my condition to myself, I wanted to excel so no one suspected I had the disease; I thought I was a success in spite of the diabetes. It's more accurate to say I succeed because of my diabetes. Staying tight-lipped about my condition deprives me of the opportunity to show others that this disease doesn't make us victims. Transparency can be a powerful testament.

Owning the disease is not easy. Tell; don't tell – the choice is yours. But one thing that is not up for debate is the need to own the *management* of your health. We don't talk much about courage, but courage is what it takes to become a successful diabetes self-manager. Your full, rich life depends on it.

CHAPTER FOUR

EMBRACING YOUR NEW NORMAL

"For a really long time,
I thought *being different*
was a negative thing.
But as I grew older,
I started to realize
*we were all born
to stand out*; nobody
is born to blend in."

———————

– Halima Aden,
First model to wear hijab on Vogue *cover*

What all people with diabetes need to learn, if they want to live a life as close to normal as possible, is how to modify their activities to account for the disease. People recently diagnosed with diabetes may be discouraged when they hear of the blood sugar monitoring, the eating restrictions and other actions needed to preserve their best health. To many, it may sound like a whole lot of stuff imposed on their routine – stuff that takes them so far out of their normal rhythm that "normal" seems lost to them forever. The truth is actually far more positive and offers much more hope.

Although the changes to routine might seem intrusive at first, these measures make it possible to head off life disruptions that come with unmanaged or poorly managed diabetes. In short, they help people with diabetes live more normal lives.

Diabetes redefines normal for anyone who has the disease. The new definition includes the critical lifesaving essentials that all people with diabetes must incorporate into their lifestyles like blood sugar tests, insulin injections, exercise and a healthy, diabetes-friendly diet. When these essentials become part of the routine, the disease produces fewer and less significant disruptions in the diabetic's life.

Diabetes also adds new dimensions to the discomfort, distress and anxieties that are part of everyone's common life experiences. Because the disease destroys the body's ability to produce insulin, people with diabetes are always at risk of having severe swings in blood sugar levels that can cause life-threatening situations.

Even so, there is no reason anyone with diabetes should have to miss out on most activities enjoyed by family and friends who do not have the disease. This kind of inclusion takes only a little extra effort on the part of the person with diabetes and the people in his or her support system. Believe me, it can be done. Those with diabetes can learn to live their own normal lives.

When I was young, nearly all of my friends knew I had diabetes. They saw me playing in the neighborhood, going to school and church and having fun with my family, just like any other guy. I always followed the rules regarding my diet, insulin administration and exercise, but I was cool about it.

At parties, for example, I ate pizza but I always carefully – and discreetly – monitored my blood sugar level to manage the carbohydrates I ingested. When I was old enough, I often had a drink at social gatherings but nursed the same beverage for the entire event. I'd duck into a bathroom to check my blood sugar or lower my head at a table to prick my finger and check my blood sugar with the glucometer on my lap. Later, when I was married, I stood behind my wife at parties to check my blood sugar.

Knowing what to do in these situations grew out of some basic concepts and behaviors I learned as a child and built upon as I aged into more freedom and responsibility. Mom and Dad set the stage early for me. When I was young, their emphasis was on two simple things: making sure I understood what my sugar baseline was and how it was reacting to my exercise, and knowing what to do when I had highs and lows while exercising. As simple as that sounds, it's not easy. The challenge for people with diabetes is learning to make tweaks along the way as they gain experience with managing the disease.

That's why Dad was so focused on exercise. If I ate a little piece of cake, for instance, he helped me learn the adjustments I needed to make with exercise to burn the extra sugar. Usually, it turned out to be a family event, like playing tennis together or going for a walk in the woods. If I had eaten the dessert without making a course correction with the exercise, Dad knew what the consequences would be. So he always insisted on doing something to counter the disease and its potential effect on me. Even after I moved out of our house, Dad would ask about my exercise during our regular phone calls.

I attended public schools in Patterson and then graduated from the University of Southwestern Louisiana with a bachelor's degree in accounting. Years later, I earned a master's degree in business administration from Norwich University. I played sports, I did other guy things with my male friends, and I dated girls.

The guys on my teams always looked out for me. If I was playing baseball or tennis and needed a Coke or something, sometimes they would even get it for me from the bag I always carried for my glove, other sports gear and snacks.

I was the team captain, so I played up to the kind of banter they gave me. If I got a great hit, one of them would say, "Hey, Armato, give me one of those Oreos or whatever you've got in there."

Where Normal Intersects Awkward

Diabetes became awkward for me only after I started dating. It was before insulin pumps came along, so I had to give myself shots. Especially when I would go out to dinner with my date – or maybe with the girl and her parents – they would recognize that I had the disease.

There is one experience I will never forget. I had been dating Anne on and off for a while, and one afternoon we started to talk about the future and our goals in life.

"I want to be an accountant," I told her, "and work for a large CPA firm."

"I know," Anne said. "You'll be great at it, too. My dream is to be a nurse or a teacher."

"Do you ever see us being together?" I asked.

She was silent for a moment. Then she answered, "Well, you know, Carl, you've got that diabetes."

When I heard those words from someone I felt really cared about me, something in my chest turned cold and empty. She was plainly saying that because I had diabetes, I wasn't good enough for her. I realized in a flash that my diabetes completely cancelled out the idea of a future together. But what hit me hardest was that she was telling me she was looking for someone who wasn't flawed liked me.

When I walked out of her house that day, I was in shock. The drive home was painful. I kept having to catch my breath, as if somebody had punched me in the gut. As I reviewed it I realized that, other than my telling her how I dealt with my disease and that there were no problems, it had never come up during our dating. Her parents knew about my diabetes. We'd all traveled to football games together. They saw me play baseball and they knew I was healthy, though sometimes I had to take breaks and get a drink or cookie out of my bag.

I'm pretty sure Anne's parents had talked to her about my diabetes. No doubt they worried about what might happen to me in the future. One way or the other, I was sure they had given her the clear message that they wanted the perfect person for her. I understand that, because I want the perfect person for my daughter. Anyway, I knew our relationship was over. After that day, we never dated again.

I dated during college, but none of those experiences ever developed into long-term relationships or to a point where it was time to discuss issues related to my diabetes. However, I remember another surprising experience with a girl I met after graduation when I was working in Baton Rouge. On my second date with Catherine, she suddenly said, "You know, Carl, I know about your problem."

"What are you talking about?" I asked. Telling her I had diabetes had never crossed my mind.

"It's all right with me," she said. "I know you're a diabetic. I did some research on you."

I was speechless. When I found my voice, I said, "I've been a diabetic almost all my life. For me, it's just a matter of adjusting diet and exercise. I've never had any problems with it, and I don't plan to have any."

"Well," she continued in a conspiratorial voice, "I have a problem, too, that I want to share with you."

I thought, *What does she mean? Is she a diabetic, too?* She said, "I've tried to kill myself."

Of course I was stunned and tried to show concern. But what dumbfounded me was her comparing my diabetes to her suicide attempt. Maybe she thought I was going to die from the disease; I don't know. Regardless, she had clearly put my disease on an equal footing with her attempting to end her life. Very quickly, I thanked her for a "great date" and told her I needed to go. We never went out again.

——— *Consider this* ———

AS A DIABETIC,
NORMAL
is whatever
YOU
make it.

Where Normal Intersects Natural

In the end, my fumbling of a football in the end zone opened the story of the love of my life.

Christi Guzzino and her family lived on the lower Atchafalaya Basin, the next street over from where we lived in Patterson. Between our houses was an empty lot where the neighborhood kids would meet to play sports. One day, the guys and girls were playing football. Angel Guzzino and I, both eighth-graders, were in the game. Angel told me her sister Christi, who was a fifth-grader, wanted to get in the game.

I looked at Christi, over on the sidelines, and shook my head. "That girl can't play," I said. "She's too little. She'll get hurt."

So Angel talked to her sister, but she gave her a different message. She said, "The only way you can play is if you tackle Carl."

In the middle of the game, I caught a pass and headed for a touchdown. I was about to cross the goal line when something hit me from behind. Christi had clipped my knees, and I hit the ground, fumbling the ball.

Christi got up, turned to her sister and said, "Can I play now?"

As we grew older, Christi and I became good friends. Besides being neighbors, we attended the same church, St. Joseph's, and we would see each other at ballgames. We used to say we would date when she got to high school, but by then I was already dating someone. I was captain of the baseball team, so Christi would come to watch the games, and we always talked afterward.

Christi and I actually did date while I was in college.

Then, when she was at University of Southwestern Louisiana and I was working in Baton Rouge, we continued to date on and off. But it was never anything serious – or so we thought.

After my experience with the girl who thought I was going to die, I had stopped dating anyone and concentrated on studying for the CPA exam. When I passed the exam, the news spread around Patterson, especially from my mom to Christi's mom. One day, Christi called to see if we could celebrate, and she drove the 60 miles from Lafayette to Baton Rouge to have dinner.

That's when our relationship got serious. After talking and teasing about it for more than a decade, we finally started dating seriously. Six months later, our talk turned to marriage, and on the day after Christmas in 1988, we were married. I'm firmly convinced that the most solid basis for a lifelong love relationship between a man and woman is friendship.

My diabetes was never an issue for Christi. We grew up together. She saw me play sports, do all the active things guys do and live the "normal" life of someone with diabetes. Not only was my disease not an issue; she never saw it as anything that would get in the way of our relationship or life in general. She never brought it up as any kind of factor that could hinder us from living fully. When she did focus on the disease, it was only to become educated about diabetes so she could be an integral part of my support system.

For us, it has always been about living a normal life together. Christi has been an angel from God in her care and compassion for me and the diabetes she helps to manage. And it all started with my fumbling a football.

Partners in This New Normal

The first week Carl and I were married, I asked myself, "Am I going to be able to do this?" His normal-looking, active life, which I'd witnessed for years, was only able to look so normal because of such careful behind-the-scenes management of the disease. This was his normal, and I was gladly making it my new normal. Still, I was scared – it was a lot of responsibility, and I didn't know how well I would handle it. After a while, I just realized that this is my life and I've got to deal with it.

So taking care of Carl became my life. Later, when we moved from Louisiana to North Carolina, away from Carl's family, he didn't have anybody else to function as his support system. It had to be me. Even though it was difficult moving away from our families, the five of us – Carl and I and our three children – have grown closer together. Just as his family of origin had a partnership, so Carl and I have a partnership. We are carrying on in much the same way they did.

I truly believe that God put me on this earth to take care of Carl so that he can do what he does now. Every day when he leaves the house, I pray, "God, please keep him safe from all danger and harm. Let people see and hear him the way he wants to be seen and heard. Keep his sugar at 120 so he doesn't have to worry." Even though I raise my kids and that's my job, too, I really feel like Carl has done so much good and he couldn't have done it without God and the support system that he has now.

– Christi Armato

HOW OTHERS SEE YOUR DIABETES

"

"No one can make
you *feel inferior*
without *your consent*."

———————

– Eleanor Roosevelt,
American activist and first lady

The label of "diabetic" can be a controversial topic in the diabetes community. Some people don't want to be called diabetic because they feel it would define them by their disease. They prefer instead to be thought of as "a person living with diabetes." For this reason, I've used the term diabetic sparingly in my writing, up to this point.

Personally, though, I think it's just easier to say I am a diabetic. I wear many labels proudly: husband, father, son, friend, leader, sports fan. Diabetic is just one more. To me, the word carries no stigma – it's part of my "normal," so I'll continue to use it. Even so, each of us is entitled to a personal opinion, so if you or your loved one prefers not to use the term *diabetic* but instead opts to use the description "a person with diabetes," that should be honored in your personal interactions.

Diabetes can have many labels attached to it – devastating, life-altering, or associated with blindness or kidney failure. When newly diagnosed people share with others that they have the disease, the reactions are predictable. Most common are "Oh, that's terrible!" "So sad!" or "Poor you." I've never heard anyone say, "What a great opportunity to adopt a healthy lifestyle!"

But I want people to know that diabetes can be an

opportunity. No, it's not the diagnosis I wanted, but I am living a richer and fuller life because diabetes forced me to be healthy, forced me to accept help when I might otherwise have been too stubborn, and forced me to cherish every moment of my life.

Living with diabetes is a journey. This journey requires continuous education for diabetics and those in their support system. It also requires trial and error, which produces success or presents opportunities to improve. Every day is a chance to maximize my health and my life.

Frankly, all people, whether or not they have a challenging disease, should live their lives with the goal of maximizing their health. I choose to consider myself lucky that diabetes forced me to adopt a healthy lifestyle.

The Things People Say . . .

My parents always treated me as Carl, not Carl-the-diabetic. As a result, I found it difficult as a child to know how to handle someone like the teacher who told me that statistically I might not make it to 40. None of those people were trying to be mean. They believed what they were saying, especially if they'd seen a loved one deal with complications of diabetes, or if they believed the statistics they heard somewhere in the days before social media became a news source for many people.

Some of the most memorable comments came from health professionals I saw. For example, when I was about 15, I went for my annual eye exam. Sitting in the exam chair, I talked with the doctor as he went through the routine of examining me.

"So, Carl," he began, "have you thought about the kind of work you want to do in the future?"

"I've thought a lot about it," I replied. "I definitely want to be an accountant."

A silence dropped around us like an invisible fog. He continued with the exam and didn't say a word about what I'd told him. Finally I prompted, "What do you think of my choice?"

There was another pause before he spoke. Then this man, a professional ophthalmologist, told me, point blank, "I think you should consider another career. You'll probably be blind by the time you're 25. I urge you to consider teaching or some other profession where you can primarily use your voice." I was devastated. The ride home with my mother was long and silent as I thought about my dreams being shattered during a routine eye exam.

During my senior year in college, I was involved in a car accident on my way back to school. I seriously injured my ankle with a compound fracture. Lying in a hospital bed in New Iberia, Louisiana, I listened to doctors who thought I couldn't hear them as they spoke in hushed tones to my parents.

"You know, I'm worried that Carl's injury just might never heal."

"You mean, because of his diabetes?"

"Sure. He'll be lucky if he walks again, much less runs."

I yelled out at them, "Oh yeah? You'd better believe I'm going to walk! I'm not only going to walk – I'm going to be running!"

My dad spoke up after he heard my outburst. He told them, "Oh, we're going to be playing tennis." In fact, when doctors finally put me in a walking cast, the first thing Dad did was take me to our town's public tennis court. He let me stand at the net and fed me balls so I could hit net shots and put the ball away with force, just like I did before the injury. My father taught me to never let diabetes prevent me from doing what I wanted. I hope I can pass that optimism and drive on to others.

Once when I was getting a cardiac checkup as an adult, a technician noticed I was sweating in the cold room. She didn't know about my diabetes, so I told her. I could tell my blood sugar was falling quickly, so I asked for a Sprite. Later when I described my history with the disease, she made a comment about how most people don't live that long with diabetes. From the way she said it, I could tell she meant to compliment me for managing my diabetes for a long time with none of the devastating damages. But even as a compliment, it was insulting.

In her defense, some healthcare professionals come into contact with diabetes only as patients seek treatment for critical problems related to the disease. Maybe their experience exclusively involves diabetics collapsing in the emergency room from uncontrolled blood sugar levels or from congestive heart failure. Perhaps they come across patients whose blindness or kidney failure is a result of poor diabetes management. If that's all they see, it may be all they know about people with the disease.

This need not be your experience, though. While it's not a diabetic's responsibility to give healthcare professionals a handle on the latest understanding of the disease, people with diabetes have opportunities to show that responsible management can lead to full, rich lives with fewer health disruptions. And why wouldn't we do this? It's in our own best interest *and* it can reshape people's view of the disease.

Stamped on My Forehead?

Everybody in my big Italian family knew I had diabetes; as I was growing up it seemed that this was the only topic they wanted to talk about with me at every family gathering. I could be getting straight A's, be on the honor roll, or be a first team all-district baseball player in high school; still, they would ask only about my diabetes.

"How are you feeling?"

"Are you having any problems?"

In their view, they were just being nice, but it made me stop wanting to talk with them.

With some people who know I have the disease, it's like it's stamped on my forehead. Somehow they're blind from seeing anything else about me except my diabetes. Trust me, people with diabetes are already self-conscious about being different; they often worry about having a problem and embarrassing themselves when they have to pause to handle low blood sugar. People may think they're helping diabetics by talking about the disease, but actually they can be pushing people with the disease away.

Even now, while some relatives and friends ask me about my career and the successes I have had, others will go straight to comments such as "How is that diabetes coming?" or "I am amazed what you've accomplished, because I know you're struggling with that diabetes." Even the phrase "that diabetes" is unpleasant. It seems to set me off from them.

Reactions like that can act as obstacles that hinder people with diabetes from achieving what they want to do in life. If you hear those comments enough, you start to wonder whether you'll ever get through to people.

You don't want to tell anyone about your disease because you might run into one of those sorry reactions. It can almost make you ashamed of having diabetes. You want to hide it, and that's a mistake.

Over the years I've thought a lot about why some people respond that way. Is it their ignorance about the disease? Are they incapable of talking about anything else? Do they just lack the depth to understand that I might not appreciate their focus on my disease rather than my interests or accomplishments? Do they really think they are being helpful and supportive? I've concluded that their reactions are more about them and less about me. I think perhaps they're afraid and unconsciously masking their fear. In their self-consciousness, they think that asking about the disease shows they're being supportive. Of course, it has the opposite effect.

People with diabetes also find it embarrassing to be called out about their disease, especially in public, as the questions usually center around compliance. In the middle of a restaurant or a family holiday party, we don't need someone asking, "Can you eat that?" People don't realize that harping on us to comply with our diet regulations can result in our *not* complying. You can have the conversation, but the education has to happen somewhere else – not in front of the whole family or out in public. Of course, this isn't only a diabetes issue; nobody wants personal issues brought up in front of friends.

My mom, for example, would jump on her brothers, who both had type 2 diabetes, about what they ate at family gatherings. It's ill advised to call out people with diabetes to the point where they will simply ignore you. Rather than telling a diabetic, "Gotcha! You're eating too much bread," or "I can't believe you're having dessert," the compassionate conversation should be held in private and should go something like this: "How can I help make sure you have the right food you need today or the right amount of carbohydrates?"

It's difficult for people with diabetes to talk about blood sugar levels with anyone but our doctors, or maybe our spouses, because it exposes how imperfect we are. No diabetic always does everything right, and we will have high or low blood sugar readings periodically even if we take all the right steps. With hard work, we'll get many normal readings, but there will also be abnormal blood sugar readings. Diabetics do not want to have to explain why these readings aren't normal or what we did wrong to cause an abnormal blood sugar reading.

―――――― *Consider this* ――――――

MEET YOUR
public relations
MANAGER:
YOU!

Even with the best intentions, people are sometimes overprotective of their loved ones with diabetes. Mom was as good as gold. She was always the caregiver when I was growing up with diabetes. She cooked the perfect meals that followed the right diet, she administered the accurate insulin injections daily, she ensured I went to all physician checkups and she was at every school or athletic event just in case I needed assistance. It was great to have her close in case I had a problem.

However, because I did have low blood sugar levels at some of these events, she feared something would happen to me. She was always overly cautious (and still is, to this day). If it had been up to her, I probably would not have been as active playing sports. She would rather I'd stayed home and close to her. Fortunately, Dad's belief in the positive effects of exercise prevailed.

Constructive Conversations to Boost Compliance

I loved talking to my father about my disease because he didn't have preconceived ideas about what was going to happen to me as a diabetic. If I had an insulin reaction or low blood sugar during a baseball game, Dad wouldn't get on my case, saying, "Carl, what the heck is your problem? You should have had a Coke!" He knew all of that was obvious and also that I didn't need to hear about it. Instead, he would say something like, "Help me understand what you think was going on so I can be more responsive if you need something." Dad would also politely ask, "Carl, can I get you some juice?"

Then, rather than becoming defensive, I'd respond, "You know, Dad, I just overdid it. I hit that triple, and then we were out; I just grabbed my glove and went straight out to the field. I probably had enough time to take a break and grab an iced tea or something. So next time, I'm not going to just run out there."

Dad always tried to have a conversation with me so he could learn. He would say, "Look, Carl, I know you've been dealing with this a long time and you're probably more of an expert than most people." Some of my doctors have learned to talk to me like that now. When I first saw John Phipps, MD, an endocrinology specialist at Novant Health, he looked at my history and noted, "Carl, you're not an endocrinologist. You're better than that because you've spent many more years than we have with diabetes. I went to college and to medical school, and I know the technology. You've experienced it the majority of your life."

Sometimes parents or others who provide support may believe that the life of a person with type 1 diabetes will someday go back to normal, but it will not. Without the proper help and management of the disease, all of the bad things people have ever read about the disease or thought would happen to a diabetic will come true. This is a tough message, but it's true.

Still, I don't think anyone with diabetes wakes up and says, "I'm not going to do today what I need to do for my diabetes." Occasionally, I think about all the people with the disease whom I've known over the years who are no longer here or who are having significant problems. I wonder: Did this happen because they didn't do what they were supposed to do to manage the disease? Or was it because they lacked the support they needed?

If some diabetics don't comply with the rules of diabetes management, somewhere in the whole support system around them, something has failed. The educational process, the tools, the training, or the know-how has been insufficient. The disease can progress sneakily. If the support group isn't helping with the different dietary needs, by the time you see complications, it's almost too late to course-correct. Say you're a type 2 diabetic who loves pizza or fast food or loves to drink, and someone in your support group is saying, "You can have a little cake" or "It's the holidays! Another drink won't hurt." Over time, a lack of vigilance will bring you down.

Diabetics need the people in their support system to be encouraging – to talk about how they can work together and deal with the disease. They need to ask questions to learn, but not to lecture. The last thing people with diabetes want or need to hear is how they ought to handle the disease from somebody who does not have the disease. If the approach from the support system is aggravating, it could send the diabetic in the wrong direction.

Instead, good supporters recognize that having the disease is difficult and they acknowledge that the diabetic is trying to deal with it. Learning to live with diabetes is a lifelong education, not only for those with diabetes but for others around them. Diabetes is a marathon, not a sprint. In short, stuff happens. You lose. You fail. Then you have to get back up and fight.

Surround Yourself With the Right Team

People often tell me how impressed they are with my career success. The truth is, my home and work environments have been behind the success all the way.

A good support team has a way of providing what you need. They give you the feeling you don't have to wrestle the disease 24/7.

I acknowledge that as the CEO of a healthcare organization it's pretty easy to have a good support system. Those whom I've asked to help me and the clinicians who are in meetings with me all know about my diagnosis. I have the luxury of surrounding myself with people who can help me if I get into trouble, but that hasn't always been the case. What was always true for me as a child is that my parents spoke to people who might be in a position to see that I needed help; they made sure these people knew what to look for and where my supplies were if they were needed. When I was older, I had those same types of conversations on my own behalf. I won't deny that those conversations feel awkward – it's hard to ask for help from others, but I have never had anyone say they weren't comfortable helping.

My wife, Christi, takes the disease on just as if she had it herself. She finds ways to support me that I don't even think about, like making me a dessert with a sugar substitute. Her support, from love to meals, has been a lifesaver. My wonderful kids, Carly, John and Tyler, understand the symptoms of the disease and offer remarkable support when I need it the most. If I'm working hard at home and my blood sugar is low, they might hear me say, "I think I'm going down," and they know exactly what to do without ever uttering a word.

If I'm giving a speech, there aren't many places I travel where I don't have someone with me who will step up and give me what I need, at the moment I need it. That way I can relax and focus on the job. There's nothing in this world like the confidence that kind of support gives me. I've never needed emergency medical attention. I never entered an ER for a diabetes-related event, because my family was always present to give the support I needed. Others might have seen those signs and said, "We need to call 911," but waiting for paramedics to arrive could be dangerous.

At times I've had a very low blood sugar level but did not want to drink the sugar a support person was offering. Once when my son John was in his teens and we'd both been active at some sport, he brought me one of those little box juices. When I'm in that state of slight decline, I don't quite know what I'm doing, so I was surprised by the drink and ended up spitting the juice all over John's white shirt. Of course I apologized – but he just smiled. That's support!

Burden or Opportunity?

Assembling the supportive team you want around you requires opening up at least to some people about having diabetes. In sharing your news, you open yourself up to a bit of overconcern – about your eating habits, your level of exertion, and so on – from a subset of people who will view your diabetes as a bit of a handicap. It goes with the territory, and I've found it requires grace (or at least tolerance) to navigate.

But when true supporters hear you have diabetes, they recognize an opportunity to help you to be your healthiest. The most skilled among them will encourage you to become more and achieve more with diabetes than you might have done without.

CHAPTER SIX

NECESSARY VIGILANCE: DIABETES DOESN'T SLEEP

"Today, our very *survival depends on* our ability to stay awake, to adjust to new ideas, to remain vigilant and to face *the challenge of change.*"

– Martin Luther King Jr.,
Civil rights leader and American Baptist minister

As diabetics, we absolutely must believe we can manage this disease. We need to have open minds to learn and confidence that we can figure out the disease. We also must be flexible and open to change when we face obstacles in our environment. Often when I speak to people with diabetes or their support team, I feel like a football coach giving a halftime locker room speech. My message to diabetics is simple: "Live the life you love. Don't let diabetes impact your life to the extent that you're coming from fear and can't have a good life."

Every person who has diabetes faces the same disease-related struggles. Whether you have type 1 diabetes from an early age or you develop type 2 diabetes later in life, the daily challenges of the disease are the same. Whoever you are – no matter your race or ethnicity, or whether you are wealthy or poor – the disease attacks the same way. What sets diabetics apart is how they respond to the disease and the challenges that come with it.

Your New Job as Monitor

A diabetic is a pancreas in action. By that I mean that when your own pancreas does not produce the insulin your body needs to regulate the sugar levels in your bloodstream, you – the person with the disease – have to do it. Your job is to behave like a healthy pancreas would automatically, excreting exactly the right amount of insulin to counter the food you eat and the stress you're under, while taking into consideration the exercise you've had.

People with diabetes must make all those judgments by collecting information about blood glucose from a sensor and pump, or glucometer, by poking a finger many times a day, and then knowing how much insulin to take to pull blood glucose down or how much food to eat to bring it up.

Managing diabetes can be tiresome work. You can never let your guard down. Others can relax, sit down and enjoy a few glasses of wine. But someone with diabetes who tries to relax by having a few drinks before bed might never wake up.

A typical man without diabetes might look forward to an opportunity to get out there with the guys on a fishing trip. But when a man with diabetes is hunting, fishing, traveling on a plane or sleeping in a tent, he's likely thinking, *How much insulin and other medication do I take with me? When are my friends going to eat or take a break in the fishing? Will they want to stay out longer than we planned?* He's supposed to be having fun, but . . . practicality prevails. Surviving the trip with no diabetes-related incident remains the bigger priority.

After I got married, my kids wanted me to go on a camp-out. Sure, it was fun, but I had to think about what might go wrong out there. During these kinds of family activities, even while playing tennis or hiking with the kids, my attention is split. I've got to think about taking care of myself, as well as others. It's like the warning they give on a plane; put on your own oxygen mask first, before helping your kids with theirs.

I've found a way to enjoy activities, but my way to relax is to have a plan. It's difficult for me to enjoy anything if I'm not prepared for what might happen, or if I don't have assistance. I might want to ride my horses in the woods, but first I have to make sure my glucose is in the normal range and my sensors and insulin pump are accurately working. I won't enjoy the ride if my blood sugar is low and I don't have something to eat.

If some friends ask me to play golf, we'll head out and while they're working on their swing, I'm checking my bag to make sure my glucose tablets aren't outdated. I confirm that I've brought enough of the right kind of food so I have no trouble when we're far from the clubhouse. Is my glucometer in my golf bag? I run through a whole mental checklist. Only then can I relax and have fun.

You can do everything right, but spontaneous situations can still arise. Suppose I'm giving a tour of the hospital to someone who prefers that we take the stairs rather than ride the elevator. The additional exercise means I have to ingest extra glucose to assure that I can stay in the right blood glucose range. So I'm suddenly on alert, watching my blood sugar all the time, stopping on the way to eat a couple of mints or glucose tablets that are always in my pocket.

Life is full of unanticipated twists, so expect the unexpected.

Anticipate Rather Than Procrastinate

Yes, things might go wrong, but diabetics also need to look for silver linings and acknowledge them. A good question to ask is this: What has working with the disease given you as a by-product that comes in handy in other ways? One of the biggest silver linings from growing up the way I did is that now I never procrastinate. In business, staying ahead of the game means you can't let things pile up; you do them now. Then, as you see unexpected things coming, you can head them off or act to allow for them.

Because I realized the potentially severe consequences of not taking precautions, I grew up quicker and matured faster than kids my age. When I planned to spend a night at a friend's house, Mom always made sure my friend's parents were prepared. I brought along the small chemistry set I used to test my blood sugar with my urine. When Mom left me with my grandparents, they couldn't give me a shot, so I learned to do it myself. I was giving myself insulin shots at age 10. After my grandmother learned she had type 2 diabetes, I gave *her* shots!

Since I was always anticipating what might happen, I often outperformed my peers in school. Planning potential scenarios was especially helpful in sports such as baseball or tennis, when I could almost see where the ball was going to go. I ran many different scenarios in my head while competing in sports, detailing what I would do if certain situations developed.

The scenario-planning discipline counted when I was earning my MBA. One example occurred when my class was divided into six teams: four student teams, a faculty team, and a computer-generated one to run a computer-simulated company. While most teams allowed the computer-generated model to determine how to manage things like inventory outages, I created a plan that predicted potential risks and solutions and manually altered our program to make the solutions I thought would be best for our company. Learning that many of the challenges presented in the scenario occurred at night, I got up several times a night to make real-time corrections. This allowed our team to be hours ahead of the competition every day.

My team members asked me how I could see when something was going to happen. I showed them that looking out for the unanticipated had a certain rhythm to it. They not only enjoyed learning that from me, but our team also ended up outperforming all the other teams. The professor told us that no one had ever beaten the computer before!

Another silver lining in diabetes is all the technology that I wear and use: the pump, the sensor, glucometers and more. All the information that I constantly process has made me very handy with technology in business. I use the same skills to look at rapid changes in the business environment. My habits of planning ahead, overpreparing, having a backup plan, educating others – they have all definitely helped to further my career.

There's also a humility that comes with recognizing my humanity. Thinking about how many times a day I monitor my blood sugar, calibrate a sensor or prick a finger, I realize how vulnerable I am. That makes me appreciate others' situations. Being compassionate is important to me. Whether someone's challenging scenario is diabetes related or not, I go out of my way to help those who might not have a plan or a backup.

Be as Diligent as the Disease

Most diabetics who pay close attention learn by trial

and error. My way is to attack the disease with the same diligence it is using to attack me. Before I got a glucose sensor, I tested my blood sugar every two hours and made insulin adjustments along the way. With the glucose sensor, I test five times a day and calibrate the sensor four of the five times for sensor accuracy. My attention to detail and commitment to dealing with the diabetes is impeccable. Even the endocrinologists who care for me are surprised when they learn how many times I test my blood sugar each day. They tell me that what I do in a month is what some of their patients do in a whole year.

People with diabetes sometimes tell me that they're struggling with the continual work of managing the disease. I respond by telling them I just try not to let the disease win. I explain that the frequent testing and calibrating are my way of course-correcting what the disease is trying to do to me. Then I always encourage them with this truth: There is no reason to believe they can't have results similar to mine.

Often people with type 2 diabetes have a mental block about dealing with the disease that is difficult to overcome. In type 1 diabetes, the pancreas has stopped producing insulin. In type 2 diabetes, the pancreas may be producing insulin, but it may not be as effective as it should be. Since the body is insulin resistant, people with type 2 diabetes need much more insulin. For them, the disease is even more of an upstream swim, requiring them to constantly take action, be their own coach, start over, learn again, do it better.

Those with type 2 diabetes have the difficult challenge of facing up to and changing the habits they developed over the many years before their diagnosis.

Let's face it – my diagnosis of type 1 diabetes at such an early age has turned out to be a silver lining because I never developed the kind of habits that are harmful to so many diabetics. Management of the disease can be much more challenging for someone who develops diabetes *after* forming the habit of eating breads and sweets and drinking sodas.

Interplay of Glucagon and Insulin

The pancreas, operating well, is an organ of precision; it carefully balances the release of two hormones that work to keep blood glucose levels within normal ranges. The pancreas secretes the hormone insulin to lower blood sugar after a meal or a drink. When blood sugar levels drop below the normal range, the pancreas secretes glucagon to raise blood sugar. This natural hormone causes the liver to release its stored sugar back into the bloodstream, where it's used as fuel.

In diabetes, this fine-tuned interplay of hormones is not carried out correctly. For this reason, people with diabetes have to help the pancreas to strike the proper balance, first and foremost through diet, exercise and carefully monitored blood glucose levels, and then through administering insulin or glucagon as needed.

In diabetics, blood sugar can drop quickly because of a missed meal or too much exercise, or because more insulin was taken than needed for the amount of food eaten. Mild or moderate low blood sugar, or hypoglycemia, can quickly become severe if not treated.

Each diabetic's reaction to low blood sugar is different. Some common symptoms include sweating, chills and clamminess; sleepiness; confusion, including delirium; shakiness; and irritability or impatience. It's vitally important that each person with diabetes knows his or her own specific signs and symptoms.

Diabetics with low blood sugar can have a seizure or lose consciousness without a quick source of sugar. If they are unable to physically eat or drink the sugar, a hormone injection from a glucagon kit can be a lifesaver.

You Think You Know the Disease . . .

When I was young, because I could always sense when I was having an insulin reaction, I never passed out from an insulin reaction or low blood sugar. But, as is common with diabetics as they mature, I started to lose the feeling that signals an insulin reaction. The first time I passed out from my disease was soon after Christi and I were married. My blood sugar was beginning to drop, and I accidentally fell asleep on our couch in Baton Rouge. Christi helped me by chopping up a glucose tablet, mixing it with water and making me drink it to get glucose in me. She called for an ambulance and she called my parents, who drove the 75 miles from Patterson in a panic. Christi's quick action with the glucose tablets worked and I didn't need to go to the hospital.

Mom and Dad had never known me to pass out. Because I'd been unconscious this time, they assumed I'd done something I should not have done, so they confronted me: "Did you exercise too much? Did you not test yourself? Did you eat just green beans for dinner and not enough carbs?"

They grilled me, and I had to remind them that diabetes is a tricky opponent. I explained that my disease was changing now that I was older and that I needed to watch it more closely because my body no longer recognized the feeling of low blood sugar that I used to sense fairly easily.

Newlywed Shakeup

Our first week of marriage I didn't know anything about diabetes-related crises, and one night I couldn't wake Carl up. I put my finger between his lips and helped him swallow some sugar water. The thought of calling an ambulance was so embarrassing, like admitting I was helpless. But I did it. I also called Carl's mother, Leona, who was a 90-minute drive away. As a 21-year-old, I was scared, but I did my best to support Carl. Two weeks later my in-laws came again to teach me how to give a glucagon shot. The glucagon shot became my best friend. I never leave home without it.

When Carl was growing up, the signs were always evident of a decline in his blood sugar, and there was always someone there to help him with it. As he became an adult, it was harder for him to tell when his blood sugar was going down. As he says, before he had a sensor, his blood sugar level could hit 30 and he could still be having a great conversation with someone even though he was just a few minutes away from passing out. That's why much of what I was facing was unknown; his mom and dad and their family had never been through the things that I was going through.

– *Christi Armato*

Incidents Are Inevitable

There will be a time – maybe today, maybe next week, maybe a month from now – when you as a diabetic will encounter something in your environment that will be different. Something will change, and your blood sugar level is not going to stay normal. If you have a hard time acknowledging it, it's as if you really are not accepting the fact that you have a disease.

Even for the person who takes all the right precautions and follows all the diabetic guidelines, something can still go wrong. Most people, including doctors, do not understand that fact; they're trained to believe that if a person with diabetes follows all the rules, everything will line up and be all right. But none of us is God. We cannot make a new pancreas or control things that make everything perfect. There's just no way to guarantee that we'll never have a diabetes-related problem.

—————— *Consider this* ——————

Just about the time
YOU BELIEVE
"I've got this,"
DIABETES
DELIVERS A
"GOTCHA!"

Most of the time, I monitor well and don't have to worry about a diabetic event. But there are times that, despite the care I take, I will miss something. Maybe I miscalculate my insulin dosage, give way too much insulin and forget to test. What can you do when something like this happens to you? You can make sure you surround yourself with people who will ensure that you come out of a low blood sugar incident.

All diabetics must find, and rely on, a person they trust who can help them when something goes wrong. For diabetic children, parents, step-parents or other relatives must step up to become that backup for them. When I was young, I had my parents, brothers and friends. Now, I have my wife, Christi, who helps me tremendously, and my children, who've learned to recognize when I need glucose tablets or something sweet to drink.

Christi learned to do many things to help me with my disease, from always cooking healthy meals to giving me glucagon injections. She sees me as the person I am, not as a diabetic. Even with all of the stress that comes with helping me manage a 24/7 condition, she has never let our lives be about the disease. She knows she might have to help me get through a diabetic event, but she never complains or looks at me as odd.

Like many diabetics, I have a continuous glucose sensor, which gives me a short-term trend of my blood sugar, and an insulin pump, which delivers doses of insulin as I need them. Before I got a sensor, there were times when I did not wake up at night because my blood sugar level dropped too low, and Christi injected me with glucagon. Without urgent glucose intake or a glucagon injection, most people in that situation have to get to a hospital in time to avoid brain damage, or worse. That's why I'm a big proponent of the insulin pump and glucose sensor. If my blood sugar level drops when I'm sleeping, my pump alarm sounds – loudly and annoyingly. I then correct and raise my blood sugar with glucose tablets, which I keep on my nightstand, in my car, in my garage and in my pocket during the day.

Trending Now

Even with a glucose sensor, I still test my blood sugar a minimum of five times a day and perhaps as many as 10 times a day if my blood sugar levels are not normal. As soon as I wake up each day, at 5 or 6 a.m., I test my blood sugar the first time; that sets the stage for what I need to do immediately, before I eat breakfast. If my blood sugar is above normal (above 100 mg/dl), I use my pump to administer some insulin right away to get my blood sugar to a normal level. I know that in the next couple of hours, it should be pretty close to normal.

A healthy blood sugar level for me is roughly between 80 and 150, so I can let myself fluctuate in that range, depending on what I do. For example, when I'm not at my desk but doing something where I exert more effort (like on rounds at a hospital), I try to maintain a level between 100 and 150. When I am scheduled to give a speech, I try to get my level up to at least 150 so I do not have to worry about having a low or getting too high, where I wouldn't be at my best.

Both physical and mental exertion can affect blood sugar levels. The stress of talking in front of a hospital board can push my blood sugar up to 200. During these meetings, I'm working to keep my blood sugar around 150 so I can be at my best. I do not always use the glucose sensor while I am working or presenting on a stage because the sensor will beep if my blood sugar level begins to drop or rises too quickly.

For instance, suppose my blood sugar level is 85 before I make a presentation. The machine would sense this as normal and not take any action, but I know I need to get the level to 150, so I eat a few sugar tablets. (Tip: Whole or dried fruit is a better-tasting alternative that can also raise blood sugar quickly.) Because I know the sensor will beep when it recognizes my blood sugar level is rising quickly to 150, I usually turn off the machine's sound during presentations.

Because I test my blood sugar regularly and review my insulin pump and sensor, I can watch the trend of my blood sugar. Mentally, I know where I started at 5 a.m., and I know the subsequent blood test results every two hours. I can track whether the level is rising steadily or quickly, or whether it has made an adjustment downward, and what the insulin impact has been during that time frame.

If you're not careful, stressful periods can drive blood sugar levels up to 200 or 250. If you eat, the food will also have an effect. So without testing or checking blood sugar every two hours and making course corrections with the insulin, your blood sugar reading could be 250 or higher within six hours, causing you to have to quickly course-correct.

Falling blood sugar levels used to make me break out in a cold sweat or get the shakes, but nowadays those signals are not as clear to me. My blood sugar level can

118 ✦ Carl S. Armato

actually fall below 70 and nobody would know it by looking at me or interacting with me. I would not know it either, and I would continue to be sharp.

At levels between 70 and 40, I'm perfectly normal. But when my blood sugar level hits 30, the reaction is quick. All of a sudden I'm struggling to recall where I am. To avoid that reaction while I am driving, I test before I get behind the wheel. Each of my family's cars has a glucometer in it, and I keep glucose tablets, snacks and drinks in every cup holder.

Even when all of that is perfect, I can still have a blip, and I have to make sure I do everything I can to safeguard against it. When I get in the car and test, if my reading is 75 or lower, I look at the insulin intake I have had the previous four hours to see what is coming in, because I know that I have to get my sugar up. If I eat three glucose tablets, I can quickly get a 30-point increase in my sugar. But if my blood sugar reading is at 30, I have to eat the whole pack of 10 tablets to get back to where I need to be. In addition, I wait until my blood sugar is normal before doing anything dangerous, including driving.

Knowing Your Numbers

The good Lord blessed me with a head for numbers. After all, I am a CPA and have an MBA. For me, keeping up with trends and utilizing technology is better than looking at a one-time glucose event. This morning, I knew where I started with my blood sugar, and I made an adjustment. I knew what I ate, and I took insulin for that. Then after about 30 minutes or an hour, I tested again to see how accurate I was.

Anyone with diabetes can do what I just described. It's not difficult. Testing takes only five seconds. Anyone can prick a finger and test blood sugar levels with a glucometer. The point is to be disciplined about it. If you don't test, you can't manage your diabetes. Without testing at least four times a day, there is no way I could have managed the disease. That is the minimum for my survival! It's all about constantly checking your assumptions, because sometimes those assumptions will be wrong. For example, if you eat pancakes for breakfast, you might guess how many carbohydrates they contain, but you could guess wrong. Maybe at lunch, you don't know whether the cook put sugar in the sauce on your food. All of these seemingly small factors affect your blood sugar, so every two hours you recheck and either adjust your insulin or add carbohydrates.

You have to be comfortable knowing that you are likely to miss and your guesses will not always pan out. You can't afford to be proud about getting it right. On the other hand, you can't beat yourself up when you're wrong. There isn't time for that; you're too busy correcting the course.

It's better to know through frequent testing that you've miscalculated or made a mistake than to run with the assumption that you're on track. An analogy might help bring the point home: Not knowing your bank account balance is worse than knowing it's overdrawn, because in the latter case you can do something about it. Similarly, not knowing your blood sugar level is worse than knowing it's 250, because without knowledge of this high reading you're unlikely to go on the attack. Likewise, if you give yourself insulin assuming you know your blood sugar level and you are wrong, it can be catastrophic. What if your blood sugar is already low before you take the insulin, and then you get behind the wheel of a car, have extreme low blood sugar and pass out? If you don't know your blood sugar, you are playing Russian roulette with insulin!

The List of Takeaways

How do you get any rest if the disease you have doesn't take any breaks? People with diabetes must be vigilant, but we can employ strategies, enforce discipline, make use of technology and enlist people who care for us to help us stand watch. With the following list of takeaways, you can begin to establish an environment that allows you to exercise control over your life in your waking hours and rest reasonably well knowing you've taken good care of the health you have:

- Test your blood sugar level often, and trace your trends.

- Make the proper corrections to keep blood sugar in the normal zone.

- Don't go without support!

- Know what can happen, and teach yourself and those in your support crew to recognize the signs.

- When planning a trip or an outing, anticipate what might go wrong, plan for it – and then allow yourself to relax.

- Acknowledge that an incident will occur someday, but don't beat yourself up when it does.

- Use your technology to your advantage so you can rest easily.

In short, take the proper precautions – and lots of readings through the day – and truly *live* your life.

What Works

Carl is so disciplined, but that's what managing diabetes takes. Every diabetic needs to realize that what works is not planning your life around the disease, but around what you can do to stay healthy.

Carl loves life and he's happy so he wants to live longer. He has a wonderful family, three beautiful children. That's what diabetics need to focus on; the people they love are the reasons that drive those with diabetes to keep figuring out what works for them to be healthy.

– *Christi Armato*

CHAPTER SEVEN

DIABETES' DARKER SIDE

"If you have a positive attitude and constantly strive to *give your best effort*, eventually you will overcome your immediate problems and find you are *ready for greater challenges*."

_____

– Pat Riley,
Former NBA coach and player

If you have diabetes, at some point you will experience difficult times. It may not always be a severe insulin reaction or crash, but there will be incidents any diabetic would rather not endure.

Diabetic shock, or insulin reaction, happens when the insulin in your system is out of balance with the amount of food you eat or the physical activity you undergo. If you're awake when the reaction starts, you should sit down to keep from falling and hitting your head, and you must get something sweet to drink. Unfortunately, in your effort to course-correct, you can also take in too much sugar; this also has consequences.

Here's a simplified explanation of what happens: Your body tells you it needs sugar. You feel so bad you will consume all of whatever someone puts in front of you – like juice or a soda – without knowing it. Once you start, you think you need more sugar, even if you've had enough. Then you rebound. Your blood sugar level can soar up above 300 mg/dl.

Sustained periods of high blood sugar (hyperglycemia) can eventually cause organ damage. Likewise, sustained lows can spell disaster. If you crash with a very low blood sugar and no one checks on you for a long period, you could undergo serious, life-threatening damage. Brain damage and death are always possibilities when a diabetic crashes. If the symptoms of hypoglycemia, diabetic shock or insulin reaction are not treated quickly, the blackout can lead to death.

Crashes can happen anytime, even if you believe you are doing everything you are supposed to do to manage your diabetes. Things happen – but this doesn't necessarily mean you're defenseless as they happen. As long as I am not sleeping, I can let my family and friends know when my blood sugar is dropping to a dangerous low. I usually say "I'm going down," and if I don't already have a sugary drink or snack handy, I tell them I need a soda. Then I sit down and try to drink enough to get my blood sugar level back up. Once my thought process is functioning again, I know to stop taking in the sugar.

But if I am asleep when my blood sugar drops below 30, I'm not able to communicate and may need a glucagon injection to get back to normal. When sleeping, I will break out into a cold sweat and start to have convulsive shakes because my body is trying to extract sugar from my muscles. I am told a crash is not a pretty sight, but I only remember what happens when I come out of it.

When I see the impact of my crash on my wife – how concerned and nervous it makes Christi – I feel terrible. In the middle of the night, she's had to give me a glucagon injection. Then she's used a cold cloth on my forehead and talked to me, telling me, "Come back, Carl. Come back!" She at times has thought I might not wake up. When I finally realize what I've just done to my wife, the first thing I do is apologize to her.

I think, *Why do I put anyone through this?* Sometimes

I beat myself up and wonder why I got married, why I had kids. I admit to moments of self-pity and regret when I think of all that my family has experienced because I have diabetes, but I'm also overwhelmingly aware I've had a blessed life. Ultimately, of course, I wouldn't change a thing.

Some people might scold a diabetic in the aftermath of a crash, usually because they are reacting from a place of fear, which I understand. When you see the effect a crash has on others, the feeling is horrible. What makes it bearable for me is that Christi never blames me for crashing. Of course she doesn't want it to happen, but she's glad she is there so we don't have to call an ambulance and go to the hospital. She says, "It's not your fault. You've got a disease. It can happen, and it does happen. That's why I'm here to help. I love you no matter what happens!"

I think Christi knows how much she is appreciated. I often tell her my success has been due to her support, as she helps me stay healthy and remains beside me through the difficult times. I simply could not do it without her. In most stories about diabetics crashing, paramedics rush to the house and treat them or take them to a hospital. For me, because Christi is in my life, the paramedics don't come, and I've had no trips to the hospital for diabetic incidents.

Nonetheless, even when you have someone there to help you, crashing is a horrible event. Recovering from a reaction is the weirdest experience I have ever had in my life as a diabetic. You do not know who you are or even where you are. You might hear someone talking to you, but it is almost like you are not there – not even in the room.

Witness to a Crash

A crash is not something you ever want to see, especially when it happens to a person you love. Over the years, there were times I wanted to film it so Carl would know what I was seeing. Sometimes, when I had to give him glucagon shots, he would regain consciousness and ask, "Why did you give me a shot?" I could tell he was upset with me. I would answer, "Because you were jumping." He'd been convulsing, but he had no idea what I was seeing. If I hadn't given him a shot, he could have died – or, at the very least, I would have ended up calling 911.

When he's crashing, Carl's not the best judge of what needs to be done. And I'm also not going to take criticism when I'm trying to help him. I guess that's how I've matured, and that's how our relationship grew. I've reached a point where I don't care what he says in the moment or in the immediate aftermath. I am going to do what I have to do to help him. But now, when he recovers from insulin shock, he thanks me and apologizes.

But I don't see the need for an apology. Diabetes is a disease you can't entirely control. You do what you can – and Carl does an unbelievable job with self-monitoring and taking precautions – but he does have a disease, and he's going to have issues. There are going to be human errors. As part of a diabetic's support team, you just have to deal with that fact.

– *Christi Armato*

Over the years, Christi has learned to recognize what is happening when I start sweating or I have a particular kind of movement. If she knows I am having a severe reaction, she immediately tries to test me or goes straight for the glucagon.

God and the Glucagon

Whenever I have to give the glucagon shot, I get on my knees and pray Carl will wake up. My faith is very important to me and I couldn't do all of this without God in my life. Anyone in this family who has anything to do with Carl gives the credit to God.

– Christi Armato

Sometimes she picks up on what my blood sugar is doing before I do. At night, she can tell by the way I am breathing if my blood sugar level is falling. She wakes me up and says, "I know you're going to test soon, but why don't you just go ahead and test now." Sure enough, when I test, my blood sugar is headed down.

Christi understands what happens when my blood sugar is either high or low. If my blood sugar is high, I am a little more irritable. If it's low, my ability to communicate changes and I may say things I never thought I said. For instance, one day when my blood sugar was low, I was trying to say that some people "had some issues." Instead, I said they "had shoes." A slip like this can signal impending trouble; but being able to read the signs gives us enough confidence to course-correct and even poke a little fun in the process.

"They've got shoes?" Christi repeated, amused. "Of course they've got shoes! I've got some shoes!"

Having someone nearby who can read these signs and steer me toward what I need to recover is invaluable. If I don't have this and I haven't monitored myself well, my blood sugar can drop through the 40s to the 30s. I start to get confused and don't realize what is happening. It's as if I drift into a place where I can't really function, and I don't know it. That is an awful feeling. When it happens to me, it takes me a while to figure out who I am, what room I am in and who is talking to me. Fortunately, with new glucose sensor technology, I know when my blood sugar is falling long before it drops too low.

——— *Consider this* ———

BATTLE

WITH YOUR OWN

FEARS,

and leave

THE REST UP TO

Something Higher.

Stacking, Rebounding, Overregulating

People ask me why I test my blood sugar so often. It's simple: I want to know my trends. If I know what the number has been the last two or three times I tested, I can see whether my blood sugar is going down or up; or, if I just ate, frequent testing tells me whether I got my insulin bolus, or an insulin surge dose, right.

Because I test a lot, I am very aggressive about keeping my blood sugar from soaring. One side effect to that is that I can actually overregulate myself, either by taking too much insulin, which can be caused by stacking, or by swinging to a high blood sugar level after a low level, which is called rebounding. Let me explain.

I always try to keep my blood sugar level between 100 and 120 mg/dl. If I test and my reading is 200, I need to get my blood sugar down. Normally it would take me three units of insulin to get the reading down to 100, assuming I was not eating any food. Let's say I check two hours later and for some reason my blood sugar is at 180. Because it hasn't gone down as much as I would like, I give myself another two and a half units of insulin, on top of the first three units I administered earlier. Because it has only been two hours, the initial dose of insulin may still be working and the second dose is stacked on top of the first. The result is that I get too much insulin and my blood sugar gets too low.

There could be several reasons my blood sugar level was still elevated. My pump site might be clogged, or perhaps the insulin entered my bloodstream more slowly because of where the site was located. Maybe I ate something and miscalculated the number of carbohydrates, and I might actually need the insulin.

I also might have made a mistake and stacked my insulin. Stacking would cause a problem because suddenly my blood sugar would start to tank, dropping quickly because of the compounding effect.

Breaks in Routine Carry Risks

Knowing your trends is important because swings in your blood sugar can happen anywhere and anytime. I used to experience a serious blood sugar low about once a month. Now, thanks to my glucose sensor, the crashes are less frequent. Without the technology, the only way to keep from crashing is to test your blood sugar often, like every two or four hours.

You are more likely to see swings in your blood sugar level if you are not in your normal routine; those are the times you have to be diligent with your blood sugar adjustments.

Close Encounter in Pre-glucometer Days

Many years ago, before glucose sensors, Carl and I were driving home to Patterson from Baton Rouge on a Friday night. I was seven months pregnant. Carl had just gotten off work and he was behind the wheel. He wasn't talking a lot. When he started taking curves at 70 mph, I warned, "Carl, you need to slow down." He wasn't answering me; then suddenly he blurted, "Christi, I can't see anything!" I had to tell him, "Take your foot off the accelerator." I took over the steering wheel and steered to the side of the road. We got his blood sugar level back on track and then I took over the driving.

Nowadays we have glucose meters and glucose tablets in every car to prevent or protect us from these events. It's so important to use them routinely, and as a matter of habit before getting behind the wheel for anything more than a short commute.

– *Christi Armato*

If your blood sugar drops while you're driving, or in a place where people do not know you are a diabetic, it can be extremely dangerous. When your mind gets confused and you can't communicate normally, people may think you are intoxicated – or even worse. Once I was driving alone on a long trip and got caught in traffic along an interstate highway. Nowadays I have a glucometer and glucose tablets handy in the center console of every car I drive, but that day they were in my bag in the back of the car and unreachable.

I began to realize my thought process was not right. Even though I was not thinking straight, I knew I urgently needed to get to an exit with a gas station to get something to raise my blood sugar. So I steered the car onto the shoulder of the interstate and took off. Before I reached an exit, a state trooper stopped me. Instead of rolling down my window to talk to the trooper, I was busy looking in my console for glucose tablets. Because he didn't know what I was looking for, he pulled his gun and told me to put my hands on the steering wheel.

Later I found out what I said and did. Somehow I was able to hit the button to roll down the window. I placed one hand on the wheel, but I was still looking for my glucose tablets. I blurted, "I'm a diabetic trying to get my glucose tablets and I need to get to a machine to test my blood." All that came out and I didn't even know I said it!

The trooper thankfully noticed I was having problems talking and understood I was experiencing a medical issue. He put away his gun, opened the car door and asked if he could help. By then I had taken some glucose tablets and my thinking was starting to come back. The officer let me get my glucometer out of the bag to test my blood sugar to see whether or not I needed any help. My sugar was at 45, so I kept eating the tablets. Because he didn't know what to do for me, he had already called for an ambulance. By the time the paramedics arrived, my blood sugar level had climbed to 102, and I didn't need their help.

I apologized to the officer. He told me I had been driving fast along the shoulder of the interstate when he stopped me. He said, "Look, Carl," – by then he was calling me by my first name – "I'm not going to give you a ticket. Just be careful, and watch what you're doing."

Sometimes when my job calls for me to travel away from home, Christi is able to go with me. But when I'm alone, I know I probably will not sleep well. Before I go to bed, I take extra precautions to get my blood sugar up to 150. Before I had a glucose sensor and trusted it, I tested myself every three hours during the night. Most of the time, I woke up on my own at these intervals; but if I had any doubt, I'd set an alarm. I'd also set an alarm if I got a bedtime reading of 115, for example, and the trend indicated it could go lower – but this alarm was set to go off in just one hour. When the alarm woke me, I'd check again so I could keep my blood sugar from falling to a point where I could not do anything about it.

Now my insulin pump and glucose sensor alarm wake me up as my blood sugar begins to fall, so I can correct before it's too late. Still, needless to say, I am much more relaxed when Christi is with me because I know we always have glucagon injections that she can give to me, if needed.

When following my normal testing routine, I am usually fine. It's when I do something out of the ordinary and fail to test that I can get into trouble. Maybe when I am on vacation, I exercise more than usual and get tired. Maybe Christi and I are attending an event and get home very late. I may have tested all through the evening, but I'm exhausted and I fall asleep without testing. Whenever I get in trouble, it is usually because I am so tired that I neglect to test.

Even though I know this, every so often I get lost in a task or a conversation that I want to finish, so I suspend the routine for what I expect will be a short time. Except sometimes it's not. Trouble can step right in and take advantage of a lapse like this.

Once I was using my tractor to cut grass, and I wanted to finish the job rather than stop to test my blood sugar. So I skipped a test. Before long, I felt unwell. By the time I tested, it was too late. My blood sugar level had dropped to 32, and I was having trouble. I ate an entire pack of glucose tablets and called Christi, who was out. She says that when she got home I told her I didn't know where I was – but I was on the tractor and it was still running.

When the glucose kicked in I was all right again. But the point is that even someone who tests as often as I do each day can miss a test and have a bad experience. Again, failure to test can spell disaster.

Wrapping up this sobering segment on the real danger that diabetes can present if not well managed, it seems fitting to hear from the people on my support team who have perhaps been challenged the most by loving someone with this disease.

A Mother's Concern

Before Carl was diagnosed at 18 months, I took him to his pediatrician because I knew something wasn't right. The doctor told me it was nothing to worry about, but I *was* worried. So I went to our family doctor and found that Carl's blood sugar reading was 800! That started our journey.

I have to give a lot of praise to his doctor; had we not had her, we would not have succeeded as we did. She said, "Leona, you have to know everything you can about diabetes." She met with me twice a day for three weeks to teach me. I took care of him for 25 years.

Sometimes taking care of the family and Carl's diabetes was overwhelming. I felt like I was just keeping my head above water. I'm thankful that my husband and I became closer and he supported me 100 percent in all the changes our family made to normalize diabetes in the house. I worried Carl's brothers might be jealous of the extra attention Carl got, but they never were. They were as much of the support for him as I was. We tackled diabetes as a family.

Carl was a sweet boy – and mischievous. If anything went wrong in my household, it was Carl. He was full of action, full of life, and still is. I had to be careful; I would sneak behind his back and tell people he was diabetic, because I was afraid that his activity level and his independent streak could create scenarios away from family where he would need support. I confess I still get a little nervous for him; I still have a mother's anxieties.

– Leona Armato

Expect the Unexpected

Carl and I choose to focus on the positive, although lots of times things aren't positive. There are some negatives, times when you feel like you don't know what to do. Because Carl's so active, it can be scary when he goes out and about on his own, fooling with his horses, taking walks; I worry about him. He gets a few hours of sleep, and he's ready to go. Carl is never going to stop trying to do more. While that can cause me some concern, it's also one of the reasons I love him.

Sometimes it's touch and go because he can't tell when his blood sugar is low as easily as he could when he was younger. Even with all the technology, you have to expect the unexpected. Recently we were catching a flight, but before we boarded the plane his pump quit working and the insulin wasn't going into him. So he gave himself a shot and tinkered with the machine the entire ride until it worked again so he could be ready for the meeting he had when we landed. That's Carl. His way of juggling amazes me, the way he figures things out on the fly. It helps that he has a little MacGyver in him.

My recommendation to the loved ones of a diabetic is that they seek help from anyone they can who can provide support. Learn from family members, medical professionals and online support groups – whatever you need to know that will enable you to help and still live your life, too. I have a goal to never call an ambulance, but I'll do it in a heartbeat if that's what Carl needs. Don't be afraid, embarrassed or defeated if that's what you need to do. Helping your loved one is all that matters when there is a crisis.

– Christi Armato

CHAPTER EIGHT

HELPING OTHERS FIND HOPE

"Our *prime purpose*
in this life is
to *help others.*"

———————

– Dalai Lama,
Tibetan spiritual leader

When I talk to people about diabetes, it is clear they want to hear the stories, not just the medical information they hear in a physician's office. They want to know how to handle the disease so they can get on with what they really want to do.

The parents of Mark, a 13-year-old I met with diabetes, told me he had decided to stop giving himself the insulin his body needed to keep his sugar in check and survive; this resulted in his spending several weeks in a hospital intensive care unit. He had an insulin pump and all the latest technology he needed, but he ate candy and sugar whenever he wanted and went days without testing or giving himself his insulin. His parents told me they had trusted him to test and give himself the insulin he needed. But he wouldn't do it. They asked me to talk to him.

When I visited Mark, after introducing myself I asked him, "How long has it been since you've tested your blood sugar levels?"

The teen shrugged. "I can't remember the last time I did it," he admitted.

"Why is that?" I asked.

"I'm tired of taking insulin," he confessed. "I just

don't want to deal with it anymore."

I nodded. "I will tell you, I got that feeling a lot as a teenager," I admitted. "I still get it today."

"Really?"

"Really. But to survive, a guy like you or me has to have a basic commitment to monitor his blood sugar and take the necessary insulin to keep it in check."

As we talked, I asked Mark what he enjoyed doing. He told me he wanted to play basketball. I listened and then said, "I played ball when I was your age. I was pretty good, too. But I was the best athlete I could be only when my blood sugar was in range. You know, if you want to be good at basketball, you need to be the healthiest person you can be."

I noticed a gleam in Mark's eye. Soon he was asking, "How did you manage your blood sugar? What happened during games?" Then came more questions, such as what to do at parties when everybody was eating pizza.

"It's OK to have a slice once in a while," I said, "but you need to understand what the pizza will do to you. You have to pay attention when you take your insulin because a piece of pizza, with all the cheese and the fat, is not going to get into your system until about four hours after you eat it. You need to check your blood sugar a couple of times when eating pizza. Before you eat pizza, check your blood sugar and take a certain dose of insulin. About two or three hours later, check your blood sugar again and take the necessary dose of insulin later. If you take it all too soon, you will have insulin working in your system, causing your blood sugar to fall before the effects of the pizza even show up. Then you will experience high blood sugar later when carbohydrates from the pizza enter your bloodstream."

That rang true for him. Mark's dad had been silent, but now he spoke up. "What happens when young people start going to parties and drinking beer?"

"When I went to parties," I said, "I didn't want to look different from anyone else. So I would get a drink, but I would carry that one drink around the whole night, and nobody knew. Diabetics have to be aware that alcohol affects them in different ways. It can make your blood sugar go up, and it can also cause you to crash."

When I left Mark and his dad, they were making plans to work together for Mark's success. I told God, *Thank You for another good talk.*

Sometimes the prospect of managing this disease seems all-encompassing. It can cause people like Mark to abandon the self-care they know they should maintain, because it seems too difficult or bothersome to do alone. Other people with diabetes can be so consumed about managing their life and their disease that they forget to develop strong relationships with others. But in both of these extremes, relationships can instill hope and lead to compliance.

Relationships fulfill us. Relationships spur us on to live more selfless lives. I like the song "You've Got a Friend in Me" because I want to be the kind of friend people can count on and I know that I need people I can count on. I've talked about how my family is my world, but I've experienced great rewards by supporting other people with diabetes. Knowing that individuals with diabetes can easily become self-absorbed, I strongly encourage them to live to serve others, which helps them stay positive and fulfilled.

At an early age I became concerned about being a diabetic narcissist, so I brought the concern up to my local priest.

"Can't I easily become too wrapped up in caring for myself and this demanding disease, Father?" I asked him. Throughout the years, I have often recalled his words.

"Carl, if you want to build good relationships and help others, it's very important for you to take good care of yourself," he answered. "If you don't make your health your No. 1 priority, how can you help others?"

I have passed that advice along to a number of people with diabetes. In fact, I find that paying attention to my care allows me to learn more helpful points I can pass along to other diabetics.

So Much Bad Press Out There

What makes it so necessary for people with diabetes to look out for each other is the widespread belief that diabetes is inevitably a crippling illness that will lead to blindness, kidney disease, possible amputations and early death. People with diabetes can be so easily influenced by such tales that many feel their prospects for leading a satisfying, healthy life are hopeless.

Educating people with diabetes about their disease is a constant battle. Many television commercials about diabetes advertise a treatment, but in the process some of them spread fearful stories – a burning sensation in the feet (neuropathy), or loss of sight in one eye, for example. Such ads you don't forget. Of course, the commercial writers follow up the negative material by including a caution to take care of yourself, but the fear has been implanted or reinforced just the same.

When I was young I wanted to learn more about my disease, so I started checking out all the books on diabetes I could find in our little public library in Patterson. Everything I read seemed to end in disaster. The examples were horrible, with pictures of people's feet turning black and discussions about amputation. The stories always ended with tragedy for the diabetic.

The more I read, the more afraid I became. Those books convinced me that I would have the same health complications other diabetics before me had experienced. I believed that having diabetes meant I would die early, before I was 40 years old.

Several times I asked my dad, "Is that going to happen to me?"

His answer was always the same and always instilled confidence in me: "Not with the way you're going to take care of yourself," he would say. "Not with the way we're going to stay ahead of this." When I showed him the terrible pictures in the books I was reading, Dad reminded me that those people may have ended up that way because they didn't take care of themselves.

"You've got to fight hard and stay ahead of it," he told me. "You've got to make sure you don't let diabetes take you down."

Because Dad was a man of faith, each of those talks ended with both of us on our knees praying in front of the couch or bed. We prayed that the actions we were taking would allow me to stay healthy and that we would do everything we could – everything that God would have us do – to stay healthy.

I want others who are dealing with this disease, particularly young people with diabetes, to know the same message my father gave to me: If they will take care of themselves, although there is no guarantee, there is hope. I titled this book *A Future With Hope* because that is the future every diabetic can look forward to, provided they manage the disease accurately and consistently.

Campaigning for What Could Be

I began talking to other diabetics about the disease when I was a teenager. During my visits to Dr. Posada's office in New Orleans, she would ask me to tell other kids about my experiences. She had a genuine interest in the field of pediatric endocrinology and wanted her young diabetic patients to learn from me. Sometimes she would know somebody who lived near my home in Patterson, and she would arrange to have the person come and talk to me. I always enjoyed the role of poster child for good diabetic care.

Over the years, as I have continued to talk with young people with the disease, I can almost always tell when they're feeling overwhelmed as they try to keep on top of all that can affect their health. I know it doesn't help to just pat them on the back and say, "It's going to be OK." These words can seem empty or dismissive to young people with the disease; they need to see that other people have figured out how to live with diabetes and deal with it successfully. They need to believe that they do not have to succumb to the disease – that despite having diabetes, they can be whoever or whatever they want to be in life. Of course, just seeing a healthy middle-aged diabetic in front of them goes a long way toward encouraging them and offering evidence of the full life they can have.

Overcomer and Encourager

I think my son Carl is amazing. I can't believe he is running a company and doing so much for others. I just wish his dad could see him today. I'm proud that Carl is trying to help other people who have diabetes. It would be easier to stay silent, but Carl never took the easy way to accomplish anything.

I used to talk with a boy with diabetes who looked up to Carl. This young man's now in college, doing great, and wants to follow in Carl's footsteps. I hope Carl's story shows others with diabetes they can run companies and enjoy their lives to the fullest.

– Leona Armato

As a healthcare executive, I have attended many presentations throughout my career about diabetes being an uncontrolled disease in our communities and across the nation and about how devastating the outcomes are for people with the disease. Typically, at banquets and galas I see moms and dads with their children watching videos showing various things that can go wrong for a diabetic. The films are shown to influence donors, but I always wish they would show other segments focusing on what goes right as a result of a regimen of disease management.

If I speak to diabetics and their families before they watch those videos, I try to prepare them for what they are likely to see and hear. I tell them about all the bad press I heard as a kid growing up. I describe what it was like when an eye doctor told me I would never be an accountant because I would go blind before realizing that goal. But then I talk about what could be. I tell them about the possibilities that lie ahead for people with diabetes, especially if they have the support they need and are willing to make the necessary life changes to manage their disease.

Consider this

DIABETES
doesn't have to
DICTATE
your
FUTURE.

WHY FOCUS ON
well-known dangers
WHEN WE COULD
PLAY UP THE POSSIBILITIES?

The last time I spoke at one of these presentations, some teens approached me and said they'd attended these events for many years, but this was the first time they'd heard a message of hope. People want to hear about the possibilities. They know the dangers all diabetics face, but they want to be optimistic about themselves, or their child, friend or loved one with diabetes. They want hope.

Once I attended a banquet in support of diabetes research with my daughter, Carly. When they started showing the video with all the tragedies, I walked out and went to the restroom to avoid seeing the negative side of the disease again. When I came out, Carly was waiting in the hallway to hug me. She has seen the other side. She knows there is hope for diabetics.

Not only do diabetics themselves need to hear positive words about the disease, but their families and friends do, too. When parents ask me to talk to their child, I know they are worried about whether or not he or she is going to live past 20 years old. That worry never goes away. My mom still checks in with me by phone every day just to be sure I'm OK. I'm a grown man but I understand her fear, so I answer or make that phone call every day to give her some peace of mind. All families need hope.

Compliance Takes Community

Sometimes the parents who want me to talk to their diabetic children complain that the kids are refusing to test their blood sugar or take insulin. Whenever I hear that, I know an unvoiced secret: It is not just the child's noncompliance; it is actually total family noncompliance. With the child sitting there, it is too awkward for me to tell the parents they are not doing their job, either. But it's true.

I worry when parents simply tell their child to comply without checking whether the child is actually doing so. The parents' failure to follow through can have dire consequences. I think families should test the blood sugar and keep logs together. A diabetic's supporters, particularly parents, need to be especially active after the diagnosis. To successfully manage the disease, people with diabetes must establish a routine of compliance from the beginning. They have to learn to test blood sugar levels regularly so they know when and how to deal with the highs and lows.

Support groups, especially parents, must always be available with the right questions and the right nonjudgmental approach. To my dad, it was second nature to be that way with me; it reflected his positive outlook on life. For other parents, developing an encouraging way with a child might take practice and patience. I know it's not easy to do, but it is so crucial for diabetics to establish a normal routine of compliance from the beginning and to believe that what they are doing will work. Diabetics and their support groups have got to address noncompliance together.

Supporting Role in Compliance

Our role in supporting a diabetic can look different, depending on our relationship to the person with diabetes. Consider the difference in approach if you happen to be a mom to someone with diabetes or if you are the wife of a diabetic. You have control over your children's compliance when they are younger, by establishing and later monitoring their routines. They need this. But the diabetic in my life is my husband, not my son. Compliance falls mostly to him, with his support people offering encouragement and action as needed.

– Christi Armato

Once a diabetic experiences a bad consequence, such as an insulin reaction or low blood sugar, it can be a learning experience leading to corrective actions in the future. The episode can lead to the realization that, with the appropriate tools and measures, "feeling better" is a matter of taking the right amount of insulin or sugar to get blood sugar back in a normal range. Sometimes behavioral issues surface, no matter how old the person with diabetes is. In such situations, parents or the support group must proactively help the diabetic learn what to do; why it is important; and how to set up detailed, disciplined approaches to dealing with the disease.

Discipline is hard, but it is needed. I do understand that in some situations parents are unable to get their children with diabetes to follow the plan, especially when the children are adults. I've had parents come to me in tears because they fear what could happen, but by then it was out of their control. I keep those families in my prayers.

Sharing Your Diabetic Experience Can Help

I also talk to adult diabetics about the disease, when the opportunity arises. For example, I once had a conversation with a man who was doing some work at my house. The man said, "I used to be a diabetic."

Experts will tell you that sometimes people with type 1 diabetes encounter what is called a honeymoon period, which is a brief remission during which the pancreas produces some insulin. It could last as long as a year but eventually ends. Maybe this man was experiencing a honeymoon period. However, he may have been a type 2 diabetic who was now medication-free because he lost weight.

Either way, I could tell the guy was not feeling well. I asked him how long it had been since he tested his blood sugar, and he told me he had quit doing that a long time ago. I gave him a glucose machine and some test strips and urged him to start using it. His blood sugar reading was above 300 mg/dl when he tested that day, and he went home because he felt unwell. Weeks later when I saw him again, he was feeling better. He said he was continuing to test and had made some diet changes. His blood sugar level was back to around 100.

In my hometown in Louisiana, I knew a person who was a teenager when his diabetes was diagnosed. By then, he had developed a lifestyle of eating and experiencing things that I never did because I was diagnosed as a toddler. He routinely ate candy bars, cake and other sugary foods. Since I was older than he was, I'm certain he'd heard me talk about the disease when I visited my family in Patterson, but he never made the commitment to manage his diabetes and, as a result, never established the habits to help him do so. He died when he was in his 40s.

After his death, my mom saw his parents, who asked about me. When she told them I was doing fine, the father talked about his son. After the son had left their house, as much as they tried to get him to take care of himself, he never got on the right path because he did not feel sick. Unfortunately, when you start to have problems, it is almost too late to correct your course, and that is what happened to this individual.

My dad used to tell me that no matter who you are, no matter what you do, no matter whether you are healthy or not, we all have something we must adapt to in life. He often noted that mine was diabetes and that I'd learned it early. Consequently, he challenged me as a child to focus on my disease and make the adjustments in my life so I could get ahead of the game. It was good advice then, and it still is.

When I talk to young people now about their diabetes, I think about how beneficial it would have been for me, at their age, to have something or someone in addition to my family to give me hope. I searched but found no hope at the library in Patterson – only those disturbing photos of people who had lost their battle with the disease. But that is changing; companies like Novant Health are making great strides in spreading diabetes education that presents a more positive picture for those who manage the disease well.

In those young people's eyes, I can see when my stories and experiences resonate. They nod their heads when I describe what happened to me as a teenager because the same thing is happening to them. They listen when I give examples of things to be aware of, like making sure to test your blood sugar before driving and always having glucose tablets in the car. What I say to them is just common sense; I share practical experiences that come from living so long with this disease. And I pray it is their message of hope.

Partnering for Health and Hope

A major obstacle that prevents the hope message from spreading widely is diabetics' own hesitation to tell others of their diagnosis and their health journey. Some people who go to support groups are not looking for hope; they'd rather sit around and complain. But most are looking for help and education. They want to share ideas that can't be learned in a physician's office. They want to hear of successes and adopt what works so they can realize their own success in managing the disease.

Diabetics learn by doing. Many will attend a class, learn about nutrition and hear about counting carbohydrates, but when they enter a restaurant they have no practical idea how to count those carbs. It's difficult to learn this from a little booklet; everyday life events don't come to you packaged and succinctly coordinated. You've got to be able to account for the curveball that life can throw you on a given day, to keep things within a normal range in order to perform.

I've had days where all the technology I wear has gone wrong. Performing well is a matter of recognizing those events and adapting quickly to take care of yourself.

Two years ago, a look at Novant Health's patient base revealed that African-American women with diabetes had a 20 percent greater chance of returning to the emergency room and being readmitted to the hospital than other patients with diabetes. Because we've changed our practices, assuring that these people with diabetes have access to medications and education, the increased risk among this group is now only 3 percent. We have learned how to influence their behavior, tracking three factors: blood sugar, blood pressure and cholesterol.

Several years ago Novant Health conducted a search and rescue program to find people who have diabetes. We tested every individual who was admitted into one of our hospitals or emergency rooms. We uncovered 6,000 cases in which people with diabetes didn't know they had the disease. Without knowing they had diabetes, they were at significant risk of complications. I'm proud that many of those patients chose to treat their diabetes and are healthier today because they were informed.

My need to come out of a total internal focus on myself was the reason I was attracted to the field of healthcare. Seeing so many with needs, I find opportunities every day to influence other people with diabetes. Beyond that personal level, through Novant Health's electronic health records in more than 500 clinics, we're able to track 100,000 people with diabetes; more than 69 percent are maintaining an acceptable blood sugar range. We not only monitor them, but the chances that they will experience negative episodes are lessened.

Novant Health outperforms all hospitals on the same data platform in terms of the care our diabetics receive.

If these initiatives produce such notable results in one health system, imagine the message of hope that could be communicated to people with diabetes if these practices were replicated across every health system in the nation. Before long, the common reaction of patients to a diabetes diagnosis could shift from horror or defeat to hope and determination that a full and fulfilling life remains ahead.

CHAPTER NINE

THE BLESSING OF EVOLVING TECH

"

"Every once in a while,
a new *technology*,
an old problem,
and a *big idea* turn into
an *innovation*."

————————

– Dean Kamen,
Inventor of the Segway

When I was diagnosed with diabetes, the only readily available way for people with diabetes to check blood sugar levels was to drop a pill in a test tube filled with urine. Times and technology have changed, thanks to research and development by medical doctors and scientists who continue to seek more answers about diabetes and – we hope – someday a cure.

From a tiny test tube for urine to more convenient test strips and glucometers, from a set daily regimen of injections to an insulin pump that gets information from a sensor, along with other lifesaving advances like glucose tablets and glucagon injections, diabetics are better able to deal with their disease than ever before.

When I was a boy, as soon as I woke up each morning, I would empty my bladder of urine from the night before. Then I would drink some water and wait to fill a little plastic cup with fresh urine. I would pour it into a little test tube, up to a marked level, and drop in a tablet. The urine would turn a color, and I would record that color on a chart.

There were four colors; based on the color, I would know my blood sugar level. The scale was from negative, which meant no sugar, all the way to 4-plus, which meant high levels of sugar were spilling into my urine. Essentially, it boiled down to two of the colors: green, which was clear, or orange, which meant I had sugar in my bloodstream.

Then there were the shots. In those days, diabetics had an established regimen of shots set by their doctor. I took a shot in the morning with 5 units of regular, fast-acting insulin and 50 units of slow-acting insulin called NPH, or isophane insulin. In the evening, right before dinner, I took a shot with 3 units of regular insulin and 20 units of NPH. My insulin dosage was set in stone and was almost never adjusted.

The only way for me to deal with fluctuations in my blood sugar level was with diet and exercise. The color scheme from the urine test let me know how much exercise I needed each day. I used that testing method from the time I was diagnosed until I was about 10 years old. My parents helped me at first, but as I got older I learned to do it myself.

Some Advances and Confidence-Builders

The problem with that old testing process was the delay. It took a while for high sugar levels in the blood to show up in the urine. The glucose measurement was not in real time; although it showed me how much sugar the urine contained, it was not an accurate indicator of how much sugar was actually in the bloodstream. Because I could not take my test tube kit to school, I was unable to test myself there to see what was going on with my blood sugar – until the debut of a special roll of tape called Tes-Tape. I carried Tes-Tape in my front pocket so I would not lose it. Yes, to me, it was that valuable.

At school I had an arrangement with the teachers. If I ever said I needed to go to the bathroom, they would let me go so I could test my urine. I remember how easy it was as I went to the boys' room, cut off a strip of tape and urinated on it. The box the tape came in had a chart with basically the same four colors as the test-tube-and-tablets process at home, and I would match the wet tape to check my blood sugar level. There was still a delay because I was testing my urine and not my blood, but at least it gave me something. Without that test, I could only rely on how I felt.

At age 10, I attended a camp for children with diabetes; it was a unique experience for me. Of course, I enjoyed being outdoors, but the camp was more about what I learned as a diabetic. When I got to camp, I was taking my normal two injections a day in my stomach and leg. After two weeks, I had learned how to give shots in my arm, my behind or anywhere. I left that camp with a lot of confidence.

Greater Dosing Freedom

Maintaining the proper doses of both types of insulin was very important. Your doctor decided the dosage, and you were not supposed to make changes.

I am thankful that Mom was there to help me when I was young. But I remember one time when she made a mistake with my established regimen of shots and accidentally gave me an increased dose of the regular, fast-acting insulin. Mom immediately panicked when she realized her mistake. The regular insulin, and not the slow-acting NPH, could have made my blood sugar drop too low, causing me to crash. This was long before I had a glucometer, so I could not just drink some orange juice to counter the effects of the insulin. That could have sent my blood sugar level sky high.

Not knowing what to do, Mom immediately called the doctor, who told her to cook me a steak so I could get some protein in my body. I will never forget that night, because I had already eaten dinner, and the doctor had her prepare me another meal of steak and baked potato. I wasn't a bit hungry, but I remember sitting there dutifully cutting that steak into bites and forcing it down. Obviously, the extra carbohydrates and protein worked. Today, in a time of constant blood sugar monitoring, fruit juice and other quick-acting carbohydrates would work (and are handier and quicker options).

Throughout college, I maintained the insulin schedule determined by my doctor. The insulin dosages did not change much, and I used diet and exercise to make adjustments to deal with my blood sugar levels. It wasn't until I had begun my career that physicians became more comfortable letting patients adjust insulin as they saw fit. Then I had the freedom and comfort of being able to change doses of insulin as I needed to.

———— *Consider this* ————

WHEN IT COMES
to technology,
KEEPING UP ON
the latest
CAN MAKE THE
DIFFERENCE.

When I was a kid, Dr. Posada would determine if my insulin dosage needed to be adjusted during my annual checkup. Back then the recommendation was for people with diabetes to visit their endocrinologist and their eye doctor once a year. If there were problems, Dr. Posada might want me to come back in six months, but usually I made annual visits to her and my eye doctor.

While there, besides a urine test I would have a hemoglobin A1C test, which gives an indication of my average blood glucose level over the previous two to three months. Hemoglobin is responsible for transporting oxygen in the blood, and glycated hemoglobin, or A1C, is formed in the blood when glucose attaches to the hemoglobin. An A1C below 5.7 percent is normal, and an A1C of less than 7 percent is usually considered excellent diabetes control.

More Frequent Exams

Since the hemoglobin A1C test showed only what had happened during the preceding three months, I really did not know what was going on the other nine months since the previous test. I continued those yearly visits until I was married, and over time I decided to see my doctors more often.

Now I get an A1C test quarterly to tell me what my blood sugar has been on average over the past three months. I see my endocrinologist every six months and my primary care physician once a quarter. For my eyes, I make an annual visit to an optometrist, who checks my eyes to update my eyeglass prescription as needed, and also to an ophthalmologist, who checks my eyes and retinas more deeply. So twice a year, I visit an eye doctor to see if there is anything to be concerned about.

Real-time Results: Real Progress

People with diabetes can check blood sugar levels nowadays with glucometers small enough to put in your pocket, but glucometers used to be much larger and usually were found only in doctors' offices. I got my first glucometer just before I went to college. It was a big, bulky machine that barely fit in my briefcase. I kept it in my apartment and would go home periodically to check my blood sugar.

Having that glucometer started a whole new evolution in the way I dealt with my disease. It meant I no longer had to carry around test strips in my pocket for urine tests. Instead of delayed results, I could know my actual blood sugar level in seconds. The new technology gave me a sense of control for the first time. I could quickly know my numbers and tell when I screwed up and when I was successful. I learned to course-correct blood sugars daily.

Not long after I moved to North Carolina in 1998 and joined Novant Health, Dr. Phipps became my endocrinologist. First, Dr. Phipps switched me to short-acting insulin and once-daily long-acting insulin. He also had me start testing my blood sugar every two or three hours.

Because the short-acting insulin ran out about every three to four hours, Dr. Phipps told me I would be giving myself so many shots that eventually I would want to use an insulin pump. And he was right. I was taking about six injections a day to keep my sugar where it needed to be. Now I have a pump and a sensor that talk to each other. The sensor measures the sugar content in the secretions right under my skin and communicates that reading to the pump.

Even so, I still test my blood sugar multiple times a day. I review my pump, sensor, glucose and insulin data to see what to adjust and at what levels. My quarterly A1C tests, along with my own blood sugar data, allow for accurate insulin pump adjustments.

The pump itself gives a steady measured dose of insulin all day, called basal insulin. Then when I eat meals, or when I'm counting my carbohydrates at meals or snacks, I take a bolus, which is an insulin dose based on anticipated carbohydrate consumption. I also have to give "correction boluses" if my blood sugar is high before a meal or to reduce high blood sugar during the day.

Technology to Give You Your Best Life

Most diabetics today have glucometers, but very few have sensors. Although sensors have been available for a while, they now have advanced capabilities, coordinating with the insulin pump. If my blood sugar starts to rise, the sensor intervenes and tells the pump to work at its maximum. If there's a low, it will reduce the insulin being delivered, tell me of the reduction, predict the result and send me an alarm.

Right now the technology is great, but it's also complicated. Even with the sensor, it takes coordination to be sure the sensor and pump will work well together. When you need it, let's say in the middle of the night, the insulin pump site might be clogged with blood or not getting insulin in it; maybe the sensor doesn't connect, or it needs to be recharged.

If people with diabetes have trouble working with the sensor, I suspect many will choose to go back to using the glucometer alone and testing many times a day. My recommendation with this, as with so many other things, is to keep fighting to make the technology work for you. Consult a diabetes educator or your physician to get help with the glucometer and sensor, but don't give up.

Today it's the sensor; in 20 years, there will be even more technology – and better technology! There is always a learning curve, but the effort of learning is worth the frustration if it helps you live your best life.

Over the years I've marveled at the increasing power of technology to put control of my diabetes into my own hands. Take innovation a bit further, and before long we may see technology capable of taking disease management out of our hands. Eventually there will probably be a closed-loop insulin pump and sensor capable of communicating with each other to deliver insulin as you need it and to control blood glucose just like a normal pancreas. I would volunteer for that!

CHAPTER TEN

DIABETES AND PROFESSIONAL SUCCESS

"*Do more than is required.*
What is the distance
between someone who
achieves their goals
consistently and those
who spend their
lives and careers
merely following?
The extra mile."

— *Gary Ryan Blair,*
Success and career coach

I remember asking my dad one day, "What would I be if I weren't a diabetic? What could I become?"

He told me, "I don't know if you'd be the same person, Carl, with the same characteristics and the same feelings, if you weren't a diabetic." His message to me then was the same as it has been throughout my life: Diabetes was not stopping me. On the contrary, it was making me be the person I am.

Dad never went overboard with it, but somehow he always helped turn diabetes into a gift, something that helped create what I would become. He showed me that the disease would shape my life in a special way. Whenever I talked about maybe working in healthcare someday, Dad's eyes would shine. He told me that because I experienced things like sticking my own fingers and taking shots every day, I would one day realize the importance of creating delightful places for people to receive care.

Though I didn't know it at the time, his counsel helped ground me in a reality of compassion for others who might be suffering in their lives. By quietly instilling in me a sense of the path that diabetes would create according to the characteristics I already had, my dad bestowed on me a sense of mission, a passion for the work I do today.

'Diabetes Won't Get in Your Way'

My parents used to tell me not to worry if people knew about my disease. They advised, "Just do the best job you can, and the diabetes won't get in your way. If you stay focused, it will be all right if people know."

But in my experience, people continued to act differently when they found out. And when I began to think about a future in business, I resolved not to tell people. I thought they would treat me like I had a handicap. Instead of seeing my capabilities, they would always see a disease called diabetes hanging over my head. I wanted to be Carl Armato, the professional, not Carl Armato, the diabetic.

That's why, for most of my professional career, I made an effort to keep my life as a diabetic private. My experience back in middle school with a basketball coach who benched me when I told him I was a diabetic had deeply affected me and led to a decision that I maintained for decades. Even the occasional instances where people found out about my disease only strengthened my resolve, because invariably they treated me differently.

In 1988, after graduating from college, I became a certified public accountant; that was also the year Christi and I were married. For several years, I worked in Louisiana at the accountancy firm Ernst & Young, rising to the level of senior tax and audit consultant. My career in healthcare began at General Health System in Baton Rouge, where I became director of finance. A few years later, I became a vice president responsible for all operational activities of First Care Physicians, a 75-member physicians group at General Health.

In 1998, Christi and I, with our young children, moved from Louisiana to North Carolina, where I first worked with Novant Health's physician divisions in Charlotte and Winston-Salem as vice president of finance and operations. Throughout this time, very few people – primarily my assistants and personal physicians – knew about my lifelong experience with diabetes.

After becoming chief operating officer of Presbyterian Healthcare in 2003, and soon afterwards president and chief executive officer, I started to tell more people that I have diabetes. These included, most importantly, Dr. Stephen Wallenhaupt, who at the time was Presbyterian's vice president of medical affairs; Dr. Ophelia Garmon-Brown, a family medicine specialist and close friend; and a few other close associates.

Not long after accepting the position of CEO at Novant Health in 2012, I began to consider opening up publicly about my life with diabetes. Then, in January 2014, I wrote a blog for Novant Health's website about having diabetes virtually all my life.

Not Easily Insurable

As my career had progressed from being a CPA and consultant to being a healthcare executive, moving up levels of authority to eventually become a president and CEO, one huge driver for me had always been life insurance. When I was a teenager, my parents bought a $50,000 life insurance policy on me with money they probably didn't have. At the time they told me that my diabetes might prevent me from getting life insurance policies.

I was shocked. My parents were trying to be positive and proactive by getting me insurance. In their mind, they were doing the right thing, but the signal it sent to me was I might never be able to get life insurance again. I remember telling them that wherever I was employed I was going to work hard and get benefits, so I would not be totally dependent on the $50,000 policy. But they always reminded me to pay the policy's premiums and not let it lapse. (In fact, that policy is still in force today, and I will never cash it out.)

Whether it was in the classroom, at a doctor's office or just with someone who did not know any better, so many times growing up I heard people say that diabetics probably would die before they reached 40 years old. My parents never said it, although I could see the fear in Mom when she heard it. But others said it, and if you hear it enough, that fear gets in your head. You know that something catastrophic could happen, even if you do the best you can. When I became a husband, father and business executive, the pressure was really on.

To provide for my family, I knew I had to work hard and show my employer that I could bring value every day. What I did yesterday was not good enough; every day I would try to outperform the previous day. The level of stress this mindset causes is heavy and difficult to describe. To wake up each day is to realize that you have so much pressure on you that you'd better get busy and try to figure out how to manage it.

At Ernst & Young, I did tax work for many corporate executives and saw that senior administrators typically received considerable benefits, including life insurance. I realized that if I could grow in a company, there would be opportunities for me to get life insurance. It also became clear that if I did not move up in the organization, those benefits I needed for my family could be very difficult to obtain.

Before long, I became a member of the American Institute of Certified Public Accountants (AICPA), which would often send notices about how to purchase life insurance through the AICPA's term life or group life plans. I cannot tell you how many times I filled out the form. I would check the box that I was a diabetic and then write a summary about how long ago I had been diagnosed and how long I'd lived with no complications from the disease. I would even get a doctor to sign off on it all. Despite those assurances, the insurers always denied me.

Father Knows Best

When I worked at General Health, a few times I considered getting out of healthcare and entering another industry where I could advance more quickly. I interviewed for a controller's job at a trucking company where the chief financial officer was near retirement. Dad thought that was a big mistake, and he was adamant. He said, "Son, I don't know how to tell you this, because you can't see it yet. But you're going to run something big one day, and I don't think it's in trucking."

Dad reiterated his message that healthcare was the path for me. He believed I could help people, not just because I had the disease but because I had interacted widely with the healthcare system. He said I would have the eyes to help workers to see how to care for patients. He said it so confidently, and he was right.

When Dad died from a massive heart attack at the age of 63, I was 31 years old – less than 10 years away from age 40 when people said terrible things were supposed to happen to diabetics. I was working at General Health, but I was not at a level in the organization to receive the benefits – specifically life insurance – that I needed for my family's security.

Dad passed away in the emergency room. In our small town in those days, cardiologists didn't have the voice they have today about what their communities need. My dad didn't receive the interventional cardiac care he needed that day, and it was absolutely devastating. For weeks it felt like I was in a dream because his death just could not be real. I had been used to talking to him almost daily, just a general phone call where he'd say, "I'm just calling to check on you because I thought you needed to hear a friendly voice." Well, I had, and now that friendly voice was gone.

I was lost. I withdrew for a year. But then I started looking back at pictures and memories. Dad had died on Jan. 4, 1996; that Christmas, my sister-in-law had given me a picture of him hugging me that I still keep near. My aunt also gave me a picture that hangs in my home, with a Bible verse that makes me think that if I can bring out even a small percentage of what he gave me every day I will be living a great life and helping others. Those tokens of remembrance helped. Still, it was a sad time. I was facing the pressure of *What's next?*

I remembered how, as I left the community to work at my first job some distance away, Dad's parting words were, "I'm so proud of you, and remember, you can always come home to Patterson if you need to." Now he no longer had my back, but by this time Christi had become a prominent, stabilizing force in my life, giving me that same reminder: "Just remember, you'll be coming home." The same faith shines in her eyes.

After my dad's death, I talked regularly with Christi's dad, Leonard "Gus" Guzzino, better known as "Papa G." He was co-owner and executive vice president of an electric company that worked mostly on big oil rigs off the Louisiana coast.

Over the years, Papa G had seen me in good times and bad, like when my sugar got low while we were playing golf. Or when we would be on vacation together and I would have a hypoglycemic reaction. But he watched my career grow and saw how I raised the kids with my wife, and he became one of my biggest supporters.

When I was getting the promotion to lead Presbyterian Healthcare in Charlotte, which was going to be a difficult job because there were many issues to resolve, I remember talking on the phone with him about whether I should face that type of stress with my diabetes. I knew what I thought, but I needed a little confirmation. I will never forget what he told me.

"Listen to me," Papa G said on the phone 800 miles away in Louisiana. "You've been living with diabetes your entire life. You're going to have it the rest of your life. Why not do what you do best and fix the things that you know how to fix and don't let the diabetes get in the way? Take the role, and fix it, and manage your diabetes like you always do." And he was that adamant about it.

———— *Consider this* ————

WHENEVER YOU
meet a challenge,
JUST SAY,
"DIABETICS EAT CHALLENGES
for breakfast."

One day as we were playing golf, I was getting ready to hit a ball when Papa G said, "Carl, I've got a question. I don't know many people who have your faith. Where did that come from?"

I started talking about my dad, what a great example his faith was, and the prayers of his that were answered over my life. I shared how many of my prayers and my family's prayers were answered through me over my lifetime and how that belief was what kept me going. I noticed that Papa G and I became closer after that.

Support at the Next Level

When I got the chance to lead Novant Health, the parent company of Presbyterian Healthcare, I knew that I was ready. I knew I could quickly bring value because the organization needed stronger partnerships with physicians, which is what I had been doing well since I was in Louisiana; I knew how to delight patients and team members.

When I was being considered for the position, I told the Novant Health board chairwoman over lunch one day that I was a diabetic and described my history. A clinician, she was amazed at all that I had done professionally while managing the disease. I came away from our conversation feeling good. As it turned out, that individual was very supportive of me with the entire board, not only during the selection process but also after I took the job.

Only a few people at Novant Health knew about my diabetes when I became the chief executive officer on Jan. 1, 2012. Obviously, senior leaders, including board members, and my caregivers were among the people who were aware, but just a few Novant Health team members were in the know.

I told my friend, Dr. Ophelia Garmon-Brown, long before anyone else at Novant Health because I trusted her. I knew she cared about me, and if I ever needed help, she would be somebody I would want to be there for me. Ophelia could figure out what to do without having to make a big deal about it. Support like that is important because sometimes you get caught up in what you are doing and need to be reminded of simple things – like that it's lunchtime.

Naturally, my physician Dr. Phipps knew of my diabetes and was very supportive. Dr. Phipps always believed that if I could apply the kind of diligence with which I handled diabetes to a big dream or Novant Health vision, we could go places. During a regular visit, I asked him a question that I had asked my dad: What would I become if I weren't a diabetic? My dad said diabetes had shaped me and my personality, and Dr. Phipps said exactly the same: that diabetes had helped create me. However, he added that he didn't know if I would have the same drive and commitment to life.

My executive assistant, Lou Ann Anderson, always provides major support for me. She knows when I need to eat and always has snacks handy in case I need them. If it has been more than two hours since I tested my blood sugar, Lou Ann will come into my office and look at me. If I'm glassy-eyed, she'll tell me I might want to check my blood sugar. Lou Ann can also tell when I've had enough office work for one day.

Even with this strong cadre of support around me, I kept the knowledge of my diabetes closely guarded, as

I'd always done. I was confident that there was a team of people in place to support me at Novant Health, but I feared that going public would hurt me more than help me. I was wrong about that. People want to help, more than I'd realized.

Time to Speak Up?

Not long after I became CEO at Novant Health, I began to think it was time for me to go public about my diabetes. The first time I brought it up, my internal communications people were worried. They asked me if I was sure I wanted to do it, since I had kept it so private for so long. They wanted to make sure I had thought it through completely.

So I decided to take my time. I waited another year, and then late in 2013, I made the decision. In January 2014, I posted the blog entry "It's Time to Merge My Job With Part of My Private Life" on the Novant Health website. It began with this paragraph:

"I've lived with type 1 diabetes for a long time. I was diagnosed at 18 months of age with juvenile diabetes. I'm confident my family and physicians would describe my disease as 'under control.' Many of you understand how challenging this can be."

My blog also announced an ongoing community outreach project related to diabetes that Novant Health would soon initiate, focusing on pre-diabetes, obesity and high blood pressure.

A lot of people were surprised to find out I have diabetes. Some of them did not realize that if people with diabetes take care of themselves, you can't just walk up to them and tell they have the disease. As usual, some people know nothing more about diabetes than an experience they might have had in their past, maybe with a grandparent. Or what they recall dates back to when there were no glucometers and people were not so actively keeping their blood sugar level under control. Perhaps all they've heard about the disease is associated with gangrene and people losing their limbs.

After that first reaction of surprise, people who read my blog were amazed to learn about my journey, specifically that someone could turn life with the disease into a positive. As I read people's comments on the blog, I was more concerned about the effort I'd expended over the years to cover up. I realized that I had hidden it too well. I'd made my pump look like a beeper or a phone. When I had low blood sugar, people might have assumed I simply was not feeling well. Even physicians were surprised. Some of it was embarrassing.

No longer hiding the disease gave me such relief. I realized that hiding my diabetes had added to the stress because so often I had needed to go somewhere to test my blood sugar while trying to make it seem like I was doing something else. But now, with my true condition known, my entire executive team is there for me if I ever need a hand, and that's nice to know.

Making It Public

In 2015, I was honored to be one of three men receiving the Father of the Year Award presented by the Charlotte Father's Day Council, in collaboration with the American Diabetes Association (ADA). Every year, the Father's Day Council recognizes men who have made their families a priority while balancing demanding careers and community involvement.

Before the event, the organizers told me who had recommended me for the award. It was some of my co-workers and others in the community who did not know about my diabetes. Naturally I was excited about the possibility of being Father of the Year. I was in the middle of the running when I met with the Father's Day Council chairwoman. She had talked with my board members, who at the time didn't know my story. Two leaders of the local ADA in Charlotte who were at the meeting also had no idea I was a diabetic, so I told them my history, about being diagnosed at 18 months and being on insulin ever since. It was a bit of a shock to them.

They asked me to be the last of the three Fathers of the Year to speak at the awards event and to tell my story. To the mothers and fathers and the many young diabetics in the audience, I said:

I think about my big Italian family upbringing, and I can only hope that I have instilled in my three children the ability to define their dreams, while having the courage to see them through. I think this is my most important role as a dad.

I reflect on how my parents never let me define myself by my diabetes. They helped me overcome the influence of certain physicians, teachers and even coaches who put limitations on me because of my diabetes – including how long I might live with such a disease. My parents encouraged and challenged me to create and follow each and every dream without limitations.

My parents helped me to write a life story that never kept me from playing sports or hanging out with friends. Diabetes didn't keep me from going to college, becoming a CPA, pursuing my MBA or becoming a healthcare leader.

I got such an unbelievable response. It was great to have people with diabetes – some of them teens – come up and tell me in tears that they wanted to know more about my journey. Some of them reached out later, to ask me to talk more about my experiences. That event not only got me energized and engaged in doing a series of similar talks; it was the impetus for writing this book.

Refusing to be Limited by 'No'

A year later, the Piedmont Triad Chapter of the Juvenile Diabetes Research Foundation honored me at the 2017 Hope for a Cure Gala in Winston-Salem. At the event, I talked about how important the word "yes" is to those of us living with type 1 diabetes, because it is a diagnosis that seems to come with a world of "nos."

Every time I heard a no – No, you can't play sports. No, you probably won't be an accountant. No, you can't pursue your dreams – I tried to listen instead to a yes, from inside me.

Yes, I did play sports. Yes, I did become a CPA. Yes, I did earn an MBA. Yes, I did become a CEO of a very large healthcare system and a healthcare leader who understands the needs of others. Yes, I learned to manage my disease even with a busy travel schedule. And yes, I even won the heart of my childhood sweetheart, Christi, and raised three happy, successful children.

That's why I leave you with one word to keep in your mind always. That word is YES! ✦

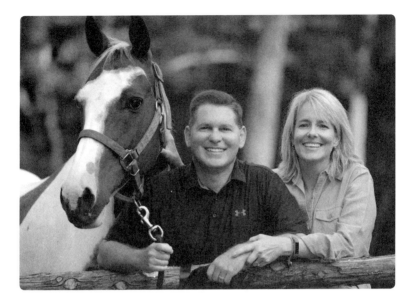

Carl S. Armato chooses to live his best life *because of* – and not in spite of – his diabetes. Diagnosed as a toddler, he thrived under his parents' determined care and their conviction that the disease would not derail his future.

They were right. Carl is president and CEO of Novant Health, one of America's largest and most respected healthcare organizations, and serves in myriad professional and civic roles, locally and nationally.

Born and raised in Louisiana, Carl lives on a ranch in Clemmons, North Carolina, with his wife, Christi, dog and horses, and enjoys frequent visits from his extended family and three children. He often speaks on diabetes-related topics, emphasizing a strong support system and active self-monitoring as keys to a healthy, fulfilling life.

This is his second book.